Cancer Etiology, Diagnosis and Treatments

Prostate Specific Antigen and Prostate Cancer

CANCER ETIOLOGY, DIAGNOSIS AND TREATMENTS

Additional books in this series can be found on Nova's website under the Series tab.

CANCER ETIOLOGY, DIAGNOSIS AND TREATMENTS

PROSTATE SPECIFIC ANTIGEN AND PROSTATE CANCER

SUDHIR ISHARWAL
AND
ZHOU WANG

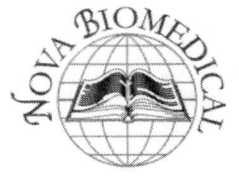

Nova Science Publishers, Inc.
New York

Copyright © 2011 by Nova Science Publishers, Inc.

All rights reserved. No part of this book may be reproduced, stored in a retrieval system or transmitted in any form or by any means: electronic, electrostatic, magnetic, tape, mechanical photocopying, recording or otherwise without the written permission of the Publisher.

For permission to use material from this book please contact us:
Telephone 631-231-7269; Fax 631-231-8175
Web Site: http://www.novapublishers.com

NOTICE TO THE READER

The Publisher has taken reasonable care in the preparation of this book, but makes no expressed or implied warranty of any kind and assumes no responsibility for any errors or omissions. No liability is assumed for incidental or consequential damages in connection with or arising out of information contained in this book. The Publisher shall not be liable for any special, consequential, or exemplary damages resulting, in whole or in part, from the readers' use of, or reliance upon, this material. Any parts of this book based on government reports are so indicated and copyright is claimed for those parts to the extent applicable to compilations of such works.

Independent verification should be sought for any data, advice or recommendations contained in this book. In addition, no responsibility is assumed by the publisher for any injury and/or damage to persons or property arising from any methods, products, instructions, ideas or otherwise contained in this publication.

This publication is designed to provide accurate and authoritative information with regard to the subject matter covered herein. It is sold with the clear understanding that the Publisher is not engaged in rendering legal or any other professional services. If legal or any other expert assistance is required, the services of a competent person should be sought. FROM A DECLARATION OF PARTICIPANTS JOINTLY ADOPTED BY A COMMITTEE OF THE AMERICAN BAR ASSOCIATION AND A COMMITTEE OF PUBLISHERS.

Additional color graphics may be available in the e-book version of this book.

Library of Congress Cataloging-in-Publication Data

Isharwal, Sudhir.
 Prostate specific antigen and prostate cancer / Sudhir Isharwal and Zhou Wang.
     p. ; cm.
 Includes bibliographical references and index.
 ISBN 978-1-61209-836-4 (softcover)
 1. Prostate--Cancer--Diagnosis. 2. Prostate-specific antigen. I. Wang, Zhou, 1964- II. Title.
 [DNLM: 1. Prostatic Neoplasms--diagnosis. 2. Early Detection of Cancer. 3. Prostate-Specific Antigen--blood. WJ 762]
 RC280.P7I84 2011
 616.99'463--dc22
                    2011004612

Published by Nova Science Publishers, Inc. † New York

Contents

Preface		vii
Chapter I	Introduction	1
Chapter II	History of Prostate Specific Antigen	3
Chapter III	Conclusion	25
Acknowledgments		27
References		29

Preface

Prostate cancer (PCa) is a disease with high incidence and prevalence. Early detection of PCa has been an area for research to decrease its morbidity and mortality. There has been significant work to detect the best serum marker for screening of it. Discovery of prostate specific antigen (PSA) revolutionized screening of PCa that was largely dependent on detection of prostatic acid phosphatase and digital rectal examination. PSA is expressed in prostate and can be detected in serum. Its level is increased in PCa along with other benign conditions. Gene for PSA is present on chromosome 19 along with other members of kallikrein family. Its structure is composed of 237 amino acids with molecular weight of 28.5 kDa. It exists in different molecular forms in serum and seminal plasma. Its physiologic function in humans is to liquefy seminal coagulum. It is used for screening of PCa with threshold value of 4ng/ml. This threshold value has low sensitivity and specificity for detection of PCa. To increase its specificity, various measurements of it such as free PSA, complexed PSA, PSA velocity, PSA density and age specific reference values has been used. Besides these measurements, several new markers have been discovered and their role in PCa detection is currently under study. PSA correlates well with high grade PCa and is a good predictor of PCa recurrence. Several leading organizations and cancer societies, based on present evidence, have published their recommendations for its use in detection and monitoring of PCa. There has been difference in opinions on its appropriate threshold value to recommend prostate biopsy and benefits on health outcomes due to its use in screening. There are ongoing trials and research, which would be helpful to scientific community in reaching a consensus for its benefits as a screening tool for PCa.

Chapter I

Introduction

Prostate cancer (PCa) is the most common noncutaneous malignancy among men in the United States[1] with an anticipated 192,280 newly diagnosed cases and 27,360 cancer-specific deaths in 2009. The medical expenditure for diagnosis and treatment of PCa was approximately $1.3 billion in 2000 [2]. Despite active efforts to diagnose and treat PCa at early stage, it is still the second leading cause of cancer-specific mortality in men in the United States [1].

PCa is generally considered a disease of elderly men. Incidence of PCa is less than 10% in age groups less than 54 years of age compared to 64% between the ages of 55-74 years [3]. Besides age; race, family history, dietary factors, androgens and environmental factors are other well-known risk factors [4-8]. Localized PCa can be treated by surgery or radiation and has an excellent outcome with minimal complications. However, treatment modalities for advanced PCa are limited and require use of hormonal therapy and eventually tumor becomes castration resistant [9].

Before the introduction of prostate specific antigen (PSA), digital rectal examination (DRE) or tissue histological examination were used as primary methods to detect PCa in patients with obstructive symptoms and enlarged prostate [10]. Prostatic acid phosphatase was used as a serum marker for PCa but by the time it increases in serum, PCa has often already metastasized to bone [11]. In 1994, the Food and Drug administration (FDA) approved PSA for PCa screening with a threshold value of 4 ng/ml, largely based on a study conducted by Catalona et al. comparing PSA to DRE for PCa detection[12].

Widespread use of PCa screening led to stage migration and there are now more cases of localized cancer rather than advanced stage PCa. Although there are clear benefits to early detection through PSA screening, medical professionals have different opinions on the survival benefits of PSA use, as a screening measure [3, 13]. In one of the recently published studies, there has been shown a modest increase in mortality benefit, however it is associated with overdiagnosis and overtreatment [14]. A major dilemma for managing this disease is over-detection and over-treatment due to increased detection of false positive and clinically insignificant tumors.

Several investigators have raised questions regarding the sensitivity and specificity of PSA for PCa diagnosis, as it has been found to also be elevated in benign prostate diseases. There are higher numbers of false positives between PSA values 4-10 ng/ml and this range of PSA value is termed as a "diagnostic gray zone". Besides a high number of false positives, the sensitivity of PSA screening is also low, as there are a significant number of men with PCa who do not have PSA values above the threshold of 4 ng/ml [15]. Several investigators have used different PSA measurements including free PSA, complexed PSA, proPSA, PSA density, PSA velocity and PSA doubling time to improve accuracy of prediction [16-19]. In addition to these PSA measurements, there are other potentially useful serum biomarkers such as prostate cancer antigen 3 (PCA3) and prostate specific membrane antigen (PSMA) for PCa detection [20, 21]. In this chapter we will discuss various aspects of PSA and its clinical use.

Chapter II

History of Prostate Specific Antigen

The discovery of PSA has been a matter of debate as various groups have claimed to detect it first. Several groups working independently and using different detectionmethods identified and named PSA differently. Later on, when immunological techniques to detect antigen in body fluids improved, it was established that all these different antigens discovered were in fact structurally similar to PSA or its complexed form [22]. In 1960, Flocks et al. were trying to develop immunological methods for PCa treatment. They isolated antigenic proteins which were prostate specific in humans[23]. Moreover, they showed that these antigens react with antibodies to agglutinate semen, suggesting expression of these antigens in body fluids [24].

In 1966, a Japanese group led by Mitsuwo Hara tried to identify antigenic proteins in semen, to serve as evidence in rape cases. They were successful in isolating a prostate specific antigenic protein and named it γ-seminoprotein[25]. This protein was later on found to be similar to PSA. In the early 1970s, Albin et al. studied antigens in normal, benign and malignant prostate. They isolated two antigens from prostatic tissue, one of which was prostatic acid phosphatase and the other that was not characterized but termed prostate specific antigen[26, 27]. Around the same time, Li et al. were trying to address the immunological basis for infertility. They observed that rabbit antibodies raised against human seminal plasma were capable of immobilizing human sperm, suggesting the presence of antigenic proteins in seminal plasma.

They isolated two antigens, E1 and E2 [28]. Later on, structural similarities were found between E1 antigen and PSA [22]. These antigens were seminal plasma specific and not prostate specific, however, they acknowledged that their technique to isolate these antigens was not sensitive enough to detect the source.

In 1978, George Sensabaugh was investigating semen of vasectomized and azoospermic males. Using gel electrophoresis of human semen, he found two unknown proteins, p30 and p41, named according to their molecular weight[29]. He used antibody provided by Li et al. to characterize these proteins and observed that p30 was identical to E1 protein. Interestingly, Sensabaugh showed that the source for this antigen was prostate rather than seminal plasma, as previously claimed by Li et al. He suggested that these antigens might be present in body fluids, but to detect these improved detection methods were needed. In 1990, with the use of improved techniques, he was able to show similarities between p30 antigen and PSA [30].

In 1979, Wang and Chu isolated an antigen from prostate using p8 antisera and named it prostatic antigen. This antigen was subsequently named prostate specific antigendue to expression in only prostate [31, 32]. In their study, they focused on purifying the antigen previously detected by Albin et al. They were able to demonstrate the expression of this antigen in malignant prostate [33]. Subsequently, Chu et al. developed an immunoassay to detect PSA and thus making it useful in clinical settings [34, 35]. Papsidero and Chu also detected PSA in the serum of men with PCa metastasis using antibody developed against PSA in prostatic tissue. This PSA differed in molecular weight from earlier detected PSA in prostate tissue due its complexed form in serum. This led to the current widespread use of PSA as a serum marker for diagnosing PCa.

In 1987, Stamey et al. were studying the role of PSA as a tumor marker for PCa using patient samples. They observed that the serum level of PSA in patients correlated better with staging and prostate tumor volume than the previously established prostatic acid phosphatase. In addition, their observation that serum PSA levels fall after radical prostatectomy suggested its use in predicting PCa prognosis[36]. On the other hand, PSA was also found to be elevated in a number of benign prostate conditions making its role in cancer detection questionable. In 1991, Catalona et al. reported that PSA could be used as a first line test for screening of PCa and was better than DRE in detection of PCa [12, 37]. Based on evidence presented by Catalona et al, the FDA approved PSA for PCa screening in 1994. Since then, several studies have been conducted to further characterize the role of PSA as a diagnostic measure for PCa and various measurements of PSA have been developed. Although several new biomarkers have been discovered, PSA is still the most widely used serum biomarker for PCa detection and prognosis.

Structure and Function of PSA-

PSA is also known as humankallikrein 3 (hK3) and is a member of kallikrein family. Kallikreins are serine proteases having enzymatic activity that can generate bradykinin from kininogens. Two distinctive type of kallikreins have been described, circulating type plasmakallikrein and glandular or tissuekallikreins, which are expressed in the local tissue environment[38]. The gene for plasma kallikrein is located on human chromosome 4 and is exclusively expressed in liver. Its major function is to cleave bradykinin from high molecular weightkininogen during blood hemostasis. Among tissue kallikareins, only kallikarein 1(hK1) has such enzymatic activity [39, 40]. Before the extensive study of the human genome, only three members of kallikrein family were known, hK1, hK2 (glandular kallikrein) and hk3 (PSA). With better understanding of human genome, 15 members of kallikrein family have been revealed. All of these genes are located on chromosome 19 and share 40-80% sequence homology with each other [41, 42]. Out of all these proteins, PSA is the major protein expressed by the prostate cells and expression of other proteins like hK2 is 10-50% compared to PSA [43-45].

PSA is produced by the secretory epithelial cells of prostate gland and periurethral glands in males [46-48]. Periurethral glands are not a major source of serum PSA, but they contribute significantly to urinary PSA after prostatectomy [49, 50]. This makes urinary PSA testing irrelevant for monitoring PCa recurrence. The epithelium of prostate glands secretes PSA directly into excretory ducts that further empty to the urethra. PSA is not specific to the prostate and expresses in non-prostate tissues including malignant breast tumors, human endometrium, perianal glands, sweat glands, breast, thyroid and placenta. However, the expression level of PSA in these tissues is much lower as compared to prostate [51-53]. PSA is a major protein in seminal fluid and its concentration varies from 0.5-2 mg/ml [51, 54]. Serum values of PSA are in the range of ng/ml in normal healthy men that is a million times less than the level of PSA in seminal fluid [37, 55].

The PSA gene is located on chromosome 19q13.4 [41] and its expression is upregulated by androgens. Promoters for PSA contain androgen responsive elements that are helpful in altering expression of PSA in presence of androgens. These promoters have also been found responsive to other steroids [56-58]. Two additional androgen responsive elements have also been reported upstream to the promoter region which may act as silencer and maintain tissue specific expression of PSA [59-62]. Lundwall et al. cloned cDNA of PSA and reported that the length of mRNA for PSA is approximately 1.5 kb[63]. A number of splicing variants of hKLK3 gene translates in to PSA like proteins but the function of these proteins has not been well defined [64-66].

In 1986, Watt et al. first reported the complete amino acid sequence of PSA. The sequence was 240 amino acids long with a predicted molecular mass of 26.5 kDa[67]. In subsequent studies, which used different methods, it was determined that PSA is 237 amino acids long with a calculated molecular mass of approximately 26.1 kDa.[63, 68].Belanger et al. using mass spectrometry determined the exact molecular mass of PSA, 28.5 kDa. They also reported that there is one N-linked oligosaccharide attached to asparagine. This oligosaccharide may be the possible reason for a difference in molecular mass calculated by earlier groups using amino acids sequence [69]. The molecular mass of PSA on gel electrophoresis was determined to be approximately 33kDa, quite possibly due to the different behavior of glycoproteins in these systems. This N- Linked oligosaccharide contributes around 7% of the molecular mass of PSA and is responsible for its binding affinity to concanavalin A [70, 71].

The mRNA for PSA translates in 261 amino acid long prepropPSA which has 24 amino acids in addition to 237 amino acids long active PSA [63, 68]. Out of these 24 amino acids, 17 amino acids represent pre region and the remaining 7 represent pro component. The pre region of prepropPSA acts as a signal peptide and directs newly formed protein to the endoplasmic reticulum (ER). In the ER, the pre region is cleaved and proPSA is packed in vesicles. These vesicles are then transported to the plasma membrane for secretion. The secreted proPSA is inactive and needs cleavage of seven amino acids from the N terminal of its activation [72, 73]. Normally cleavage occurs between amino acids arginine and isoleucine resulting in the formation of the active form of PSA. However, sometimes cleavage occurs between leucine 5 and serine 6 resulting in a truncated form of PSA. This truncated form is termed as [-2] pPSA as it contains two extra amino acids and is catalytically inactive. Further truncated forms of PSA, with one, four or five extra amino acids have also been reported. These truncated forms of PSA have been shown to be elevated in PCa tissues and serum [74, 75]. Activation of PSA by digestion of bonds between arginine and isoleucine can be done by enzyme trypsin. In the prostate gland, this activation is done by humankallikrein 2, which has trypsin-like activity [76, 77]. PSA activation can also be done by human kallikrein 4, which is also expressed in the prostate along with PSA [78].

Over the years, several structural models for PSA have been suggested. These models were primarily based on the amino acid sequence of PSA and its homology to other serine proteases [79-81]. Recently, the crystal structure of PSA bound to monoclonal antibody 8G8F5 has been reported. This antibody supposedly provides stability to this structure. The catalytic site of PSA is composed of amino acids His57, Asp 102 and Ser 195 [82]. Due to this composition of catalytic site of PSA, it is included in the serine protease family that includes trypsin and chymotrypsin. Enzymatic activity of PSA is similar to chymotrypsin and is different from the other kallikreins, which show trypsin-like activity [67, 83-85]. Similar to other members of kallikrein family, PSA structure also contains a kallikrein loop. This loop stretches from amino acids 95-101. The amino acids of the kallikrein loop limit access to the substrate-binding site of PSA, providing it substrate specificity compared to chymotrypsin. The active site of PSA contains three hydrogen bonds, one between His57 and Asp and two other between His57 and Asp102 [82]. Zinc is a well-known regulator of physiologic function of PSA and has been thought to inhibit its enzymatic activity[86]. The zinc interacting surface of PSA is composed of amino acids 25, 78, 91,101,229. These amino acids align with each other to form a binding site for zinc [82].

Various molecular forms of PSA have been discovered in the human body. PSA circulates in blood, either free or complexed to protease inhibitors. Approximately 80-90 % of the PSA which enters the blood is catalytically active and rapidly conjugates with α1- antichymotrypsin (ACT) and α2-macroglobulin (A2M)[87, 88][16]. Small amounts of serum PSA are also complexed to α1-protease inhibitor, which shares homology to ACT [89, 90]. The level of ACT present in serum is significantly higher than PSA. This suggests that the remaining 20-30% of PSA, which circulates as free PSA, is not capable of forming complexes with ACT. This covalent binding of PSA to protease inhibitors prevents substrate from binding to catalytic sites and thus makes it enzymatically inactive [84, 91, 92].

Although ACT is expressed along with enzymatically active PSA in prostate, less than 1% of PSA has been detected in complexed form[93, 94]. In seminal plasma, most of PSA is free except less than 5%, which is bound to protein C inhibitor [95, 96]. 70-80% of the free PSA present in seminal plasma is active and the rest has been shown to have internal clipping, making it inactive[70, 84]. These internally clipped forms of PSA maintain their size as these fragments remain attached by internal disulfide bonds and comigrates with intact PSA on SDS-PAGE [67]. There are various sub-forms of free PSA in serum: BPSA, proPSA, intact but inactive PSA (iPSA)[97, 98]. BPSA is mainly mature native PSA with internal cleavage at amino acids Lys182 and Lys145. Its level has been found to be elevated in patients with benign prostatic hyperplasia (BPH) [99-101]. proPSA is truncated form of PSA in which there are extra 1-5 amino acids. These forms are more resistant to activation by both trypsin and hk2 [74, 75]. It has been found to be elevated in prostate tumors compared to BPSA and is predicted as a better marker for PCa than free PSA [102]. iPSA is formed when mature, active PSA is proteolysed and becomes inactive. This form has also been predicted to be helpful in distinguishing malignant prostatic diseases from benign prostate conditions [103, 104].

To distinguish different forms of PSA, various assays have been developed which rely on recognition of its epitopes by monoclonal antibodies. Various groups have used a number of monoclonal antibodies and the International Society conducted several workshops for Oncodevelopmental Biology and Medicine to better define the epitopes of PSA. In 1997, in the third workshop, an agreement was reached that there are mainly six epitopes of PSA out of which one is free PSA specific, one has cross reactivity with hk2 and the remaining four can be recognized in its free as well as ACT complexed form. Recognition of epitope groups 1, 3, 4 and 5 are conformation dependent, as these are composed of nonlinear amino acids. When ACT forms a complex with PSA, it completely masks epitope group 1 and makes it unavailable to antibodies. This forms a basis to distinguish complexed PSA from its free form. Antibodies developed against free PSA failed to detect its complex form with α2 macroglobulin [88]. α2 macroglobulin is substantially larger in structure compared to PSA and is believed to mask all of its epitopes [84, 105].

In 1994, the FDA approved PSA assay for screening of PCa and the upper limit for PSA in healthy persons was set at 4ng/ml. Its approval was mainly based on evidence presented by Catalona et al., using a Tandem-R assay for PSA developed by Hybritech Corporation [106]. Subsequently, several studies showed that different methods to assay PSA give different values even with same samples. These differences raised a need for standardization of assays for PSA [107-112]. In 1997, the National Committee of Clinical Laboratory Standards, in an attempt to resolve inter-assay variability, published recommendations for the standardization of PSA assay [113]. Shortly after this, the World Health Organization (WHO) adopted recommendations of several studies and issued the International Reference Preparation (IRP) 96/670 for total PSA and IRP 96/668 protocols for free PSA measurement [114-116]. The method to determine molecular mass of PSA, recommended by WHO, was different from that used by Hybritech Corporation. WHO adopted use of mass spectrometry and determined the mass of PSA as 28.5 kDa compared to approximately 34 kDa determined by Hybritech Corporation using the Lowry total protein method. This difference in mass resulted in 20% increase in molar absorption coefficient; 1.84 as determined by WHO compared to 1.42 as previously determined by Hybritech Corporation. This 20% increase in molar absorption, resulted in 22% difference between cutoff values of PSA, for prostate biopsy, by these two methods. Previously, the cut off value for normal PSA 4ng/ml was determined using Hybritech method which was equivalent to approximately 3.1ng/ml determined using the WHO method. In spite of all these efforts to standardize, there is still variability present among different assays. This generates a need to reach a consensus, so that a single universal value can be suggested for PCa biopsy [117].

In the human body, PSA by virtue of its enzymatic activity has been known to hydrolyze semenogelinI, II and fibronectin. This activity is helpful in liquefaction of seminal coagulum after ejaculation [118, 119]. Liquefaction of semen decreases semen viscosity and increases sperm motility. PSA has also shown to hydrolyze insulin like growth factor binding protein-3 (IGFBP-3), which is a binding partner of insulin like growth factor-1 (IGF-1). Cleavage of IGFBP-3 makes it inactive and it can no longer bind to IGF-1 [120, 121]. IGF-1 acts as a mitogen in PCa growth [122, 123]. Clinical correlation has been shown in patients with PCa and decreased level of IGFBP-3 levels [124]. In a recent in vivo study, Niu et al. showed that PSA could mediate proliferation of castration resistant prostate cancer by enhancing transactivation of androgen receptor via a coregulator ARA70[125]. PSA has also been suspected to play a role in bone metastasis. It has potent osteoblastic activity which may be due to its activation of transforming growth factor-beta, modulation of osteoblast cell surface receptors or cleavage of parathyroid hormone related peptide, an inhibitor of osteoblastic activity [126-128]. On the contrary, PSA has also been linked to antiangiogenesis. It has been reported that PSA inactivates fibroblast growth factor-2, vascular endothelial growth factor and cleaves plasminogen to generate peptide fragments with angiostatin like activity [129]. This inactivation of pro angiogenic factors and generation of antiangiogenesis factors suggest its antitumor activity. Clinical use of PSA as a tumor marker for PCa is well established and we will discuss it in detail in following sections. PSA is also expressed by breast cancer but its role in diagnosis or follow up has not been well established [130-132]. Enzymatic activity of PSA is being tried for therapeutic use in PCa. Several antitumor prodrugs have been developed which can be specifically cleaved by enzymatic activity of PSA and thus rendered active in prostate tissue [133-135]. This can be a very promising field to explore for new drug treatment options for prostate confined tumor.

PSA as a Diagnostic Marker for PCa

PSA was discovered in the 1960s and 70s, but it took another decade for multiple studies to suggest its role in diagnosis of PCa [34, 136]. At the time of discovery, there was not sufficient data to justify its use for monitoring or diagnosis of PCa. In 1986, the FDA approved use of PSA for the monitoring of PCa in already diagnosed patients, largely based on evidence provided by Ercole et al [11]. In 1991, Catalona et al reported that PSA can be used for screening of PCa and is better than DRE, used for this purpose at that time [37]. However, there were several studies, which reported that PSA elevation can also occur with age, inflammation of prostate and BPH in addition to PCa, making its role suspicious for diagnosis of PCa[36]. In 1992, American cancer society recommended its use as a part of annual physical examination. Two years later, mainly based on a multicentre study conducted by Catalona et al, the FDA approved use of PSA for screening of PCa with a threshold value of 4ng/ml for prostatic biopsy[12]. Since then, there has been a lot of work to evaluate its role as a diagnostic serum biomarker for PCa.

PSA levels in serum are a million times less than its level in prostate and seminal fluid[137]. This difference is mainly due to tight compartmentalization of PSA by ductal structures of the prostate. When there is disruption of normal prostate architecture, serum levels of PSA increase due to leakage in blood. This disruption of prostatic architecture can occur in various conditions including BPH, prostatitis, PCa or any kind of injury or manipulation like biopsy, massage, or digital rectal examination of prostate [11, 54, 138]. Besides prostatic diseases and manipulation, riding a bicycle, strenuous physical activity and ejaculation also have been shown to affect serum levels of PSA [139-142]. Hormone levels and drugs like 5α reductase inhibitors also alters PSA levels in serum [143, 144]. Physiologic serum level of PSA becomes detectable during puberty due to increase in serum testosterone level [145] and increases with enlargement of prostate volume with age[146]. Alterations of serum PSA level by all these conditions makes it less specific for diagnosis of PCa and make its elevation in serum difficult to interpret.

After the introduction of PSA screening, there was initially increase in incidence of PCa until 1992, and after that incidence declined gradually [147]. This initial increase in incidence was explained due to the screening effect of PSA and diagnosis of previously undiagnosed cases. PSA screening has also led to decrease in incidence of advanced stage tumor and increase in incidence of localized PCa resulting in stage migration and greater prevalence of localized stage in population [147, 148]. PSA took control from its predecessor DRE and was shown to be a better screening tool for diagnosis of PCa[12]. However, in a randomized control trial, DRE led to detection of 17% of cases, which were undiagnosed by PSA screening alone [149]. Multiple studies observed that, screening using both methods is better than either of them alone [12, 150]. Based on PCa patients studied by several studies, it has been observed that, cases diagnosed by DRE are high grade and at advanced stages compared to those diagnosed by PSA [149, 151, 152]. Thus, PSA and DRE are complementary to each other and use of both is recommended for screening of PCa in clinical settings.

For effective treatment of cancer, there is a need for a test that not only diagnoses the cases but also predicts risk of having it in future. The role of PSA in predicting development of PCa was first evaluated by Stenman et al. in 1994. However, this study was limited by having only a small patient group of 44 [153]. Subsequently, a larger prospective study conducted by Lilja et al. concluded that, in an age group of 44-50 years, a single PSA test can predict risk of development of PCa later in life [154]. Ulmert et al., based on their case control study, reported that PSA tested at or before age 50 is a strong predictor for development of PCa up to 25 years later [155]. This ability of PSA to predict risk of developing cancer, decreases with increasing age mainly due to increase in PSA value due to higher number of BPH in older males[156]. Furthermore, several studies concluded that higher value of PSA is associated with higher relative risk for development of PCa in future with a lead-time of 5.5 years [157, 158]

Use of PSA for screening of PCa has positively affected diagnosis and monitoring of PCa. Prostate biopsy driven by increased levels of serum PSA above threshold has led to detection in 27-44% of cancer cases [151, 159, 160]. However, there is still a large percentage (50-70%) of population who has increased value of serum PSA and is false positive for PCa. This put these patients at risk for unnecessary biopsy, financial burden and psychological trauma. The numbers of false positives are higher in PSA ranges of 4-10 ng/ml, mainly because of the prostate specific nature of PSA rather than cancer specific and thus increased by various prostate conditions other than PCa. This range of PSA (4-10ng/ml) is thus termed as diagnostic gray zone. There have been various attempts to improve PSA specificity for PCa in this range of serum values. In order to resolve this issue, a number of measurements of PSA like PSA density, free PSA, complexed PSA, PSA doubling time and age adjusted PSA reference values have been tried to make PSA a better diagnostic serum marker for PCa.

Free and complexed PSA- As already discussed in this chapter, PSA circulates in blood as complexed form which is bound to protease inhibitors or an enzymatically inactive, unbound form termed as free PSA. Total PSA refers to both free and complexed form. Currently available assays can easily detect both forms in the serum. In 1993, Christensson et al. first found that value of free serum PSA was lower in patients with PCa as compared to patients with BPH [87]. Subsequently several studies supported this finding, suggesting role of free form of serum PSA in increasing specificity of PSA for PCa[153, 161, 162]. Luderer et al. showed that free PSA was able to detect additional 31% cases over total PSA, when used in patients with total PSA in the range of 4-10 ng/ml [163].In the same year, Catalona et al. confirmed these findings with their study and reported the percentage of free PSA is an independent predictor of PCa[164]. This specificity can further be increased by excluding men with prostate volume more than 50ml, as with the increase in prostate volume, there is increase in percentage of free PSA [165, 166]. Catalona et al. reported that using a cut off value of 23% free PSA for prostatic biopsy, it can prevent 31% unnecessary biopsies in patients with prostate volume greater than 40ml and a cut off value of 14% would have prevented 76% unnecessary biopsy in patients with prostate volume less than 40ml[164]. In another study by Catalona et al, they observed that a cut off level of 25% for free PSA detected 95% of cancer and eliminated need for 20% unnecessary biopsies [152]. In this study they also predicted the risk of PCa, based on percentage of free PSA in serum and reported that PCa risk is 8% in patients with free PSA more than 25% to 56% when free PSA is in between 0-10%. Catalona et al. also evaluated role of free PSA in patients with total PSA value of 2.6-4 ng/ml and found that it has a positive role in diagnosis of PCa in these patients [15]. Based on all this data, FDA approved use of percentage free PSA for PCa diagnosis.

As already discussed in this chapter, there are three subforms of free PSA- proPSA, BPSA and iPSA. It has been shown by Mikolajczyk et al. that precursor form of PSA;proPSA is associated with PCa while BPSA is associated with BPH [99, 102]. They reported that, majority of proPSA was a truncated form of PSA containing 2 extra amino acids at its N-terminus. Peter et al, using mass spectrometry reported presence of other truncated forms of PSA with 4, 5 and 7 extra amino acids at its N terminal end [167]. However their study included patients with total PSA between 6900-8500 ng/ml of total PSA that is much higher than the range of 4-10 ng/ml where specificity of total PSA is less. Later, with the development of antibodies to different truncated forms of PSA, [-2]pPSA was found more specific form to be detectable in PSA range of 4-10 ng/ml[75]. [-2]pPSA has been demonstrated in PCa tissues of patients using immunostaining[102] and the possible reason is its resistance to activation by hk2, thus, being more stable than other forms [75]. Expression of BPSA is higher in BPH patients and its role in diagnosis of PCa is not the same as of proPSA but it might play a role in diagnosis of BPH. The role of iPSA, which represents minor variants, has not been fully understood yet and further research is needed. Thus, free PSA and proPSA plays a role in increasing specificity of PSA in the patients with total PSA values in diagnostically gray zone (4-10 ng/ml).

Complexed forms of PSA with protease inhibitors were also thought to improve specificity of PSA based on their higher serum levels in patients with PCa[168]. In a multicentre study, it was observed that complexed PSA has higher specificity in diagnosing prostate carcinoma compared to total PSA [169]. Complexed PSA has higher specificity compared to total PSA but has similar specificity to the percentage of free PSA [170, 171]. It eliminates the need to measure both free and total PSA to determine percentage of free PSA and thus, it would be more cost effective. All these studies show that use of percentage free PSA and complexed PSA is very promising in increasing specificity of PSA. Increase in values of free and complexed PSA with age and interassayvaribilities are the kind of issues which need to be resolved before reaching a consensus to set a threshold value to recommend prostate biopsy based on the values of free or complexed PSA.

PSA velocity – PSA velocity was first reported by Carter et al. while longitudinally studying the levels of PSA in a non screening clinical setting [172]. PSA velocity can be defined as the rate of change in serum PSA over a period of time. As serum levels of PSA depend on the volume of prostate [36, 173], with increase in prostate volume there should be an increase in level of serum PSA. Based on this, rate of change of PSA seems to be a better indicator of growth of prostate compared to a static value of PSA. It has been reported that PCa growth rate is much more than BPH [174]. So PSA velocity for PCa should be different from BPH. Carter et al. in 1992, compared PSA velocity in frozen serum samples among patients with PCa and BPH, using persons with healthy prostate as controls [172]. In this study, they observed that PSA velocity of 0.75ng/ml/yrcould differentiate between patients with or without PCa. This rate of change of PSA was found in 72% men with PCa while only 5% patients with BPH showed this kind of change. This observation has been further supported by several studies, which also report that using PSA velocity of 0.75ng/ml/yr has a specificity of more than 90% for prostate carcinoma [175-177]. However, physiological variability between the measurements of PSA in same individual at different time points remains an issue. In addition to this, change in PSA over a short period of time is also a concern regarding its specificity for PCa[178, 179]. This physiologic variability is between 10-30% of PSA level [180, 181] and can be addressed by using PSA measurement over a long period of time with multiple intervals. The minimum follow up time requirement to establish PSA velocity specific for PCa, was determined to be three measurements over a period of 18 months [176, 179, 182]. These all studies used patients with PSA value in the range of 4-10ng/ml. Although a few studies have showed that PSA velocity is promising in diagnosis of PCa below PSA value of 4ng/ml [183], there is a need for more conclusive evidence. Despite all these evidences in support of use of PSA velocity to increase specificity of PSA in diagnostic gray zone, Vickers et al. in their systemic review observed that there is not enough evidence to support its use in clinics. They concluded that its use does not provide any benefit over total PSA for prediction of PCa[184]. These contradictions show that there is need for further studies to conclude its diagnostic role.

PSA density- The concept of PSA density was introduced by Benson et al. in 1992 when they used ratio of serum PSA to prostate volume to specifically differentiate between PCa and benign prostatic disease. They determined prostate volume by transrectal ultrasonography in a population of 533 men and predicted that inclusion of PSA density in nomograms may be helpful in predicting PCa in diagnostic gray zone[185]. Subsequently, multiple studies further established this relationship of PSA density to PCa[186, 187] and a threshold value of 0.15 was suggested to differentiate cancer from benign disease of prostate in the PSA range of 4-10 ng/ml [188]. However, the role of PSA density is not well established. It has been reported that using PSA density of 0.15 for diagnosis would have missed 30-50% of cancer in this PSA range [12, 189]. As calculation of PSA density includes prostate volume in its measurement, different detection rates of PCa by biopsies might be a function of prostate volume. Uzzo et al. confirmed this in their study that patients with negative biopsies have larger prostate volume compared to patients with positive biopsies. They concluded that men with higher prostate volume need more biopsies as tumor volume relative to prostate volume may affect its diagnosis [190]. In addition to prostate volume, variability in amount of PSA secreting epithelium and shape of prostate, to calculate volume of prostate, are hurdles in its application for diagnosis of PCa [191, 192]. However its role in rebiopsy for PCa after initial negative biopsy but still high PSA, has been suggested[193]. In addition to questions about its sensitivity for PCa, invasiveness and cost to use transrectal ultrasound, also limits its clinical use. Catalona et al. found similar detection rates using percentage free PSA compared to PSA density. They recommended the use of percentage free PSA instead of PSA density [194].

Age specific reference PSA values- In 1993, Oesterling et al. correlated serum PSA levels with age and prostatic volume, which in turn was also correlated with patient age. In this study, they postulated that instead of using a single PSA value for all age groups as an indication for prostate biopsy, age specific values should be used. In their study, they proposed use of serum threshold PSA values of 2.5ng/ml for 40-49yr, 3.5ng/ml for 50-59 yrs, 4.5ng/ml for 60-69 yrs and 6.5ng/ml for 70-79yrs old age groups[195]. These age specific reference values were projected to provide more sensitivity in younger age group by having cut off values less than 4ng/ml and higher specificity in older age group, with higher serum PSA values, more often due to BPH. Morgan et al., who reported that age specific reference PSA values could be used to increase sensitivity and specificity of PSA for diagnosis of PCa, further supported findings of their study. They also pointed out that serum PSA values in black men are higher compared to white males and need different age specific reference values. If these same reference PSA values were used for black population then 40% of PCa cases would be missed [196]. These recommendations were surrounded by controversies as Catalona et al. reported that use of these cut off values would result in up to 60% under detection of PCa [194]. Crawford et al. reported that use of age specific reference values along with DRE achieved higher specificity but at the same time there was a decrease in sensitivity leading to lesser detection of PCa. They supported continual use of PSA value 4ng/ml along with DRE for detection of PCa[197].

New biomarkers for PCa diagnosis- PSA though widely used for screening, diagnosis and staging of PCa, has several shortcomings. Low specificity of PSA for PCa detection results in high false positive rate, leading to overdiagnosis and overtreatment. In PCa prevention trial (PCPT), it was reported that there is no PSA threshold value at which it has both high sensitivity and high specificity for PCa and cancer risk is present at all values of PSA[198]. Thompson et al. also reported that even advanced PCacould be detected below serum PSA value of 4ng/ml [199]. As discussed earlier in this chapter, none of PSA derivatives except free PSA is recommended for use to detect PCa. Hence, there is urgent need for new biomarkers for PCa detection and staging with high sensitivity and specificity. With the advancement in proteomics, high thoroughput techniques and understanding of human genome have resulted in discovery of new biomarkers; however their clear benefit in PCa detection, staging and prognosis still remains to be established.

Human Kallikreins- With the understanding of human genome 15 members of human tissuekallikreinshas been discovered. Out of all these members expression levels of eight members have been found to be elevated in PCa. Among these members use of KLKs 2- 4, 11-14 and 15 have been implicated as biomarkers for PCa[41].

hK2 (humankallikrein 2)- As discussed earlier, hK2 shares 80% structural homology with PSA. It has been shown to be expressed in prostate tissue, where it serves as an activator of PSA due to its trypsin like enzymatic activity[72] The expression level of hK2 has been shown to be lower in prostate tissue and body fluids compared to PSA [43, 51]. In the past years, its low level in body fluids had made it difficult to measure and limited its application in PCa detection. With the advancement in purification techniques and monoclonal antibodies, it has become easy to assay it in persons suspected of suffering from PCa [200, 201]. Expression level of hK2 has been found to be elevated in PCa tissue and more specifically correlate with tumor grade and stage. Immunohistochemical studies have shown that its expression level is more in higher Gleason grade tumors compared to low Gleason grade PCa[202-204]. Application of hK2 has also been tried to improve specificity of PSA for PCa. Ratio of hK2 to free PSA has been shown to have better specificity for PCa in the range of 4-10ng/ml total PSA while there is no significant improvement in using ratio of hK2 to total PSA [205, 206]. Its role has also been implicated in predicting pathological stage and to determine eligibility for repeat biopsy[207]. There is suggesting evidence that hK2 and its ratio to free PSA are better indicator for repeat biopsy for diagnosis of PCa[208].

Other Kallikrein markers- hK4 is expressed mainly in basal epithelial cells of PCa and its expression level has been found to be elevated in PCa cells [209]. Use of hK11[210], hK14[211] and hK15[212] has also been suggested.

Prostate specific membrane antigen (PSMA)- PSMA is a membrane glycoprotein that is expressed in prostate epithelial cells. It is a type II integral membrane protein with a molecular weight of 100kDa. It has two domains, one small intracellular and large extracellular domain[213, 214] Expression of PSMA has been demonstrated in PCa tissue using monoclonal antibody MoAb7E11-C5[21]. In the immunostaining slides, it was observed that PCa tissue stain darker as compared to benign tissue, which was slightly or moderately stained [215, 216]. Several studies have shown high expression of PSMA in the serum of patients suffering from PCa compared to healthy patients [217, 218]. There has been development of radioscintiscanning scan(ProstaScintTM) using antibody raised against PSMA to detect metastasis of PCa[219]. ProstaScint scan has shown to be more sensitive and accurate than currently used imaging studies in detecting local lymph node invasion[220]. All these evidence provide strong support for its role as biomarker for PCa however it is still evolving.

PCa antigen 3 (PCA3) – It is also known as DD3 (Differential Display Code 3). PCA3 was discovered due to its differential expression in PCa tissue and benign prostatic tissue. PCA3 gene encodes several RNAs that differ from each other due to alternative splicing and other posttranscriptional changes. These RNAs do not translate into proteins and are believed to regulate gene expression [20, 221]. Expression of PCA 3 was found to be elevated in PCa tissue compared to normal prostate [20, 222]. Its expression level was 140 times more in PCa tissue compared to BPH [223]. Prostate cells shed during the first void urine after DRE of patients and this forms basis to check for RNA of PCA3 in urine to reveal PCa. Diagnostic accuracy for detection of these RNAs in urine and prostatic fluid had been compared and found to be similar [224]. This makes it highly convenient to test for these RNAs, eliminating need for prostatic biopsy. There has been recommendation protocol for performing DRE before testing PCA3 in urine [225, 226]. In order to determine how effective screening marker PCA 3 is, several studies determined its area under the receiver operator characteristics curve (AUC) and found it to vary from 0.66 to 0.87 [226, 227]. AUC of PCA 3 was higher as compared to PSA, suggesting that it is a better marker for detection of PCa [224, 226]. PCA 3 is a promising marker for PCa; however, its utility for PCa detection and prognosis needs further evidence, before recommending its use in clinical settings.

Other new biomarkers- With the advancement in technologies there has been discoveries of several new biomarkers for PCa like Insulin like growth factor and binding proteins, early PCa antigen, α-methylacyl-CoA racemase,

TMPRSS2:ERG, Transforming growth factor β1 and interlukin 6 to name a few. Discussion of all these biomarkers for PCa is beyond the scope of this chapter and has been reviewed in several articles [228, 229].

PSA and PCa recurrence- In addition to its clinical use in diagnosis and monitoring of PCa, PSA has also been used to detect failure of therapy for PCa. For the tumors localized to prostate, radical prostatectomy has been a reliable treatment option for several years. In radical prostatectomy, removal of complete prostate is done which is major source for PSA in human body. This results in a decrease in PSA level to undetectable in serum in cases where tumor is localized to prostate. In these cases any elevation in levels of PSA after prostatectomy suggests failure of therapy, though the serum PSA level to define therapy failure varies from 0.2ng/ml to 0.4ng/ml [230, 231]. In patients who undergo radical prostatectomy, but serum PSA levels does not fall to undetectable level, are considered to suffer from systemic disease [232, 233]. Sharp rise in PSA level in these patients suggests metastatic disease, while gradual increase in PSA value indicates local recurrence [233]. Defining PCa recurrence after treatments other than radical prostatectomy like radiotherapy, brachytherapy, is much more difficult as PSA does not become undetectable after these treatments. However, American Society of Therapeutic Radiology and Oncology (ASTRO) panel defined it as PSA levels greater than absolute nadir plus 2ng/ml or current nadir plus 3ng/ml at call or 2 consecutive increase of 0.5ng/ml back dated [234]. Median time for PSA recurrence has been measured and varies from 8-16 years [235, 236].

Several pretreatment variables like Gleason score, stage of PCa, pretreatment PSA value, DNAploidy, race, tumor volume, prostatic acid phosphatase, angiogenesis, p53, p27 and ki67 have been studied to predict PCa biochemical recurrence [237-249]. In order to predict PCa recurrence after therapy, Partin et al. developed an equation that was helpful for PCa in stage T2b, c. According to this equation, relative risk for PCa recurrence Rw is; Rw = (0.061×sigmoidal transformant of PSA (PSA_{ST}) + (0.54×postop. Gleason sum) + (1.87×specimen confined)[240]. Bauer et al. also developed a biostatistical model equation, according to which relative risk of recurrence Rr = exponent [(0.51×Race) +(0.12×PSA_{st})]+(0.25×postop. Gleason)+ (0.89× organ confined)[250]. Several other nomograms and equations have also been developed to predict PCa recurrence using preoperative characteristics of patient [249, 251, 252]. These nomograms and equations have been useful in predicting PCa recurrence, however with the stage migration in recent years their use has become less practical. After failure of therapy for PCa, rate of change of PSA predicts the growth of PCa and several studies have tried to relate PSA doubling time with progression of PCa. It has been reported that in patients with doubling time more than 3 months, PSA doubling time is related with PCa death in a continuous manner[253]. Increase in PSA after PCa recurrence is linear with time and follows first order kinetics [254, 255]. Addition of other characteristics like Gleason score for tumor and time to PSA recurrence, make PSA doubling time a better predictor of PCa deaths [235, 236]. After recurrence, various imaging methods like bone scan, CTscans, indiumcapromabpenditide scan and transrectal ultrasonography have been used to define the area of its recurrence [256, 257]. However, the decision on the single most effective modality depends on other factors and is debatable. There are currently many treatment options available in clinics for PSA recurrence of PCa like salvage radiotherapy, salvage radical prostatectomy, salvage cryotherapy and hormonal therapy. Although PSA doubling time predicts progression of PCa, treatment options depend on individual patient characteristics and kind of therapy received by him initially. PSA has been useful in predicting PCa recurrence and its doubling time correlates well with mortality due to PCa and thus serves as a marker to predict and monitor PCa recurrence.

Guidelines for screening of PCa- In order to promote evidence based clinical practice leading organization in urology have laid down a few screening guidelines to effectively detect patients with PCa. These recommendations are very helpful to clinician in making decision about potential candidates, method and interval of screening. These recommendations try to make these screening criteria standardized and universal. For effective implementation of these recommendations, screening measures should be valid, sensitive and specific so that patients can trust these methods. These recommendations are based on available evidence and try to address concerns of patients and clinicians have regarding PCa screening. Several leading urological associations and societies have described following effective screening measures.

American Urological Association (AUA) guidelines- AUA recommends that for early detection of PCa, all men above 40 years old with at least 10 yr life expectancy should be offered screening for PCa. This PSA testing at 40 years serves as baseline PSA value for the comparison with future elevation in PSA level and further testing should be based on this value. Patients, who wish to be screened for PCa, should be offered both PSA and DRE. These patients should be explained about potential benefits and risks of PCa screening. Patients should know general interpretations of this screening and about physiologic changes in PSA level like its increase with age. During interpretation of the values of PSA, other factors like prostatitis, BPH, trauma, drug intake and prostate manipulations, should also be considered. AUA does not recommend a single cut off value of PSA for making decision to biopsy. It recommends that when making a decision to biopsy other factors like race, family history, prior biopsy history and other health issues, should also be considered. Patients found positive on PCa biopsy should be explained about all the treatment options with their risks and benefits. Further information about AUA guidelines for prostate cancer can be found at (http://www.auanet.org/content/guidelines-and-quality-care/clinical-guidelines/main-reports/psa09.pdf).

United States Preventive Services Task Force (USPSTF) recommendations- USPSTF found convincing evidence in favor of screening for PCa by PSA. It states that PSA is more sensitive for screening of PCa compared to DRE. It recommends use of single PSA value 4ng/ml and points out that use of lower PSA values will increase false positive cases. In its risk assessment, it categorizes patients with positive family history, older age and African American as high-risk patients. It finds insufficient evidence to determine accurately if there is any health benefit for the cases detected by screening over the ones that are diagnosed by clinical detection in patients less than 75 years. USPSTF assessed that harm of PCa screening outweighs benefits achieved by screening in patients older than 75 yrs and thus discourage PCa screening in this age group. If there is mortality benefit is found due to screening then screening interval of 4 years may have same benefits as achieved by annual screening. It recommends PCa screening on individual basis after discussion with the patient on benefits and harms of it[258]. American academy of family physician also agrees with the recommendation of USPSTF for screening of PCa[259].

American Cancer Society (ACS) recommendations- ACS recommends use of PSA and DRE for screening of PCa. In its guidelines, it advises health care professionals to offer screening to all 50 years old men with average risk and who have life expectancy of at least 10 yrs. This conversation should start at 45 years in high-risk patients (African American, positive family history for early PCa). In patients with multiple first-degree relatives suffering from PCa before 65 years of age, screening is advisable even at 40 years of age. Benefits and limitations of PCa screening should be discussed with all the patients before offering to test for PCa. Once screening is started, patients should be tested annually with both PSA and DRE. In case, patient leaves this decision to his physician, he should be tested in absence of any contraindications.

However, due to insufficient evidence ACS does not recommend routine testing for PSA [260].

American College of Preventive Medicine (ACPM) - ACPM reviewed medical literature available prior to July 2007. They observed that PCa screening has potential to decrease morbidity and mortality due to PCa; however, this observation remains unproven in absence of sufficient evidence to support it. Major limitation of PCa screening is number of false positive and false negative cases resulting in overtreatment and underdetection. ACPM does not recommend routine screening for PCa. It advises clinicians to discuss benefits and limitations of PCa screening thereby helping them to make informed decision[261].

All these leading health organizations have put forth their recommendations based on the literature available on PCa screening. Due to the conflicting results on benefits of screening, there is not a universal guideline applicable in all clinical settings. These organizations agree that PCa screening can decrease morbidity and mortality due to PCa; however, there is different opinions on its routine use in general population. Health care professionals should identify high-risk population based on their character-istics like race, age and family history and appropriately counsel about PCa screening. These recommendations encourage clinicians to provide inform-ation about limitations, benefits, alternatives and interpretation of screening. In brief, health care professional should discuss every aspect of PCa screening with candidate patients and help them to make informed decision based on all the evidences we have so far, for the screening of PCa.

Controversies regarding its use as screening method- Since its discovery and widespread clinical use as a screening tool, PSA have been surrounded by several controversies. These controversies still persist even after two decades of considerable efforts to better characterize PSA as a tumor marker for PCa. There are several concerns regarding its use such as appropriate threshold value for prostatic biopsy, age for starting screening and most importantly mortality benefit achieved by its application in screening. An ideal screening measure should have high specificity and sensitivity to correctly identify every patient with the disease. Specificity of PSA has been a major concern for its application as it is prostate specific rather than disease specific.

PSA is 60-70% specific at its widely used threshold value of > 4ng/ml [262, 263] resulting in the detection of a significant number of false positive cases. To increase its specificity, age specific reference values of PSA were projected for clinical use [195]. However, these values lead to decrease in overall sensitivity thereby underdetectingPCa patients [194]. Besides specificity, sensitivity of PSA is also determined by its threshold value for prostatic biopsy. It has a sensitivity of 70-80% at 4 ng/ml with positive predictive value of 31-54% [263]. This results in the underdetection of PCa and thus, depriving significant number patients from benefits due to early detection of PCa. Catalona et al observed that decreasing threshold value to 2.6 ng/ml would increase its sensitivity, resulting in to detection of additional 22% clinically significantPCa cases [15]. This lowering of the threshold value would also result in increased detection of prostate confined tumors with lesser tumor volume [264]. However, there is the concern that it would lead to overdiagnosis of clinically insignificant PCa which might not progress [265].

The sensitivity and specificity of PSA suffers from verification bias. This verification bias develops as all the patients undergoing screening does not undergo biopsy to correctly determine there true status. Punglia et al. tried to measure the effect of verification bias on specificity and sensitivity of PSA for PCa, using a mathematical model[266]. Correction for this bias resulted into increase in area under receiver operating curve, suggesting an improvement in its discriminatory power for PCa. They also supported decrease in threshold value of PSA to 2.6ng/ml arguing that it would result in significant improvement in sensitivity at the expense of little decrease in specificity. Another support to this argument came from PCPT. PCPT was free from any verification bias as all the patients enrolled in this study were encouraged to have prostate biopsy regardless of their PSA values [199]. It showed that PCa can be detected at all the serum values of PSA and increase in PSA value is associated with increased risk of having PCa. Their study favors decrease in threshold value of PSA to increase detection of PCa. In 2004, Stamey et al. argued against the use of PSA for screening of PCa, based on the results of their study [267]. In this study, they concluded that correlation of PSA with PCa has decreased since its initial use in 1983. Now it correlates significantly with size of prostate and weakly with cancer volume. Their study tried to establish correlation between PSA value and high grade PCa and did not emphasize on prediction ability of PSA for PCa. However, their study started a debate whether PSA era has come to an end or not. In subsequent studies it was established that PSA values still correlates well with the risk of advanced disease and biochemical recurrence after prostatectomy [268, 269]. Based on these results Freedland et al. stated that the "PSA era is alive and well" in the United States.

Numerous questions have been raised in previous years regarding benefit on health outcomes due to screening of PCa. In order to justify vast expenditure and the unfavorable effects of screening [270], there should be some mortality benefit to continued screening. Until recently, there was a lack of sufficient data to accurately estimate mortality benefit due to PCa screening. There was only one randomized clinical trial in which mortality data was published and it reported 62% reduction in mortality due to screening of PCa using PSA with threshold value of 3ng/ml [271]. This study was limited due to differences in follow up period in different groups, low compliance rate and failure to compare experimental group with control during analysis. Recently, two large studies, European Randomized Screening of Prostate Cancer (ERSPC) and Prostate, Lung, Colorectal and Ovarian cancer screening trial (PCLO) published their results on the effects of PSA screening on mortality due to PCa[14, 272]. PCLO trial was conducted across 10 centers in United States in a population of age group 55-74 years. These men were randomized to experimental and control group. Experimental group was screened by PSA for 6 years with PSA threshold value of 4ng/ml and DRE for 4 years. The median follow up time for both groups was 11.5 years. There was a 22% increase in detection of PCa in screened population compared to controls; however, there was no significant difference in mortality between these groups. The possible explanation for modest increase in detection rate of PCa by screening is, due to widespread use of PSA testing in United States, 52% of the control group underwent PSA testing compared to 85% of experimental group. This led to comparison between higher screening (85%) group to lower screening (52%) group. The lack of mortality benefit might be due to short follow up period as only highly aggressive PCa cases progresses quickly to death, high (4ng/ml) threshold value of PSA for undergoing biopsy. In this trial, 44% of the participants had already underwent PSA testing which ruled out the potential PCa cases who would have detected by screening in trial and only 30% men who had PSA elevation >4ng/ml underwent screening, so true status of all these persons was not determined. According to Dr Patrick Walsh, "Because this study was poorly planned and executed, the results of this trial are worthless when giving advice to a healthy man about impact on death from prostate cancer if he undergoes intelligent screening with PSA, a prompt biopsy when an abnormality is found and effective therapy"[273].

ERSPC trial was also started around same time in seven European countries with larger group of patients. The core group enrolled for study was 55 to 69 years old. In majority of centers, threshold value for PSA was 3ng/ml with screening interval of 4 years and median follow up time 9 years. There was approximately 71% improvement in cancer detection rate along with 20% mortality benefit in the screened population compared to control group. However, in order to prevent a single PCa death, 1410 men need to be screened and 48 men need to be treated. ERSPC showed that PCa screening has modest mortlity benefit at the expense of overdiagnosis and overtreatment. One limitation of this study was lack of uniform guidelines to biopsy for PCa, across all the centers. In order for prostate cancer screening to be successful, Dr Walsh advises not to overdiagnose older patients who are less likely to have survival benefit and avoid overtreatment of younger patients with low tumor volume[274]. Results of these studies leave us in ambiguous situation and to make a decision in support of or against screening of PCa is highly complicated. The best course of action for now is to make a shared decision by providing information to the patients and considering cost effectiveness, overdiagnosis, overtreatment and limitations of mortality benefit.

Ongoing trials and research- In order to clear this ambiguous situation there is clearly a need for more studies. The ERSPC and PCLO studies are currently ongoing and will publish their findings after increased follow up in future. In addition to these trials, the Prostate Cancer Intervention Versus Observation Trial (PIVOT) in the US [275] and the Prostate Testing for Cancer and Treatment (PROTECT) trial in the United Kingdom[276], are currently being pursued and hopefully, would be able to answer all these questions regarding screening of PCa.

Chapter III

Conclusion

PSA has been a reliable tool for screening of PCa for the past two decades. Its introduction revolutionized detection and monitoring of PCa patients. Its journey, since its discovery, has been controversial, first about its discovery and then its clinical application and survival benefit due to it. There is consensus that its use has led to increased detection and stage migration of PCa. However, there is no serum PSA value at which we can effectively rule out presence of PCa. It remains a good predictor of presence of high grade PCa detection and PCa recurrence. There is difference in opinions about mortality benefit achieved by its use in screening and this requires further studies to reach an agreement. However in the absence of a better alternative, it is still most widely used serum marker for PCa detection and prognosis prediction and would continue to be.

Acknowledgments

We thank Drs Laura Pascal and Prabhpreet Singh, for critical reading and insightful discussion.

References

[1] Jemal, A; Siegel, R; Ward, E; Hao, Y; Xu, J; Thun, MJ. Cancer statistics, *CA Cancer J Clin* Sudhir Isharwal[1] and Zhou Wang[1], 2009, 59, 225-249.
[2] Penson, DF; Chan, JM. Prostate cancer. *J Urol.*, 2007, 177, 2020-2029.
[3] L. Ries DMaMDea, SEER cancer statistics review: SEER Web site http://seer.cancer.gov/csr/1975_2005/.
[4] Kalish, LA; McDougal, WS; McKinlay, JB. Family history and the risk of prostate cancer. *Urology.*, 2000, 56, 803-806.
[5] Henderson, BE; Ross, RK; Pike, MC; Casagrande, JT. Endogenous hormones as a major factor in human cancer. *Cancer Res.*, 1982, 42, 3232-3239.
[6] Cotter, MP; Gern, RW; Ho, GY; Chang, RY; Burk, RD. Role of family history and ethnicity on the mode and age of prostate cancer presentation. *Prostate.*, 2002, 50, 216-221.
[7] Steinberg, GD; Carter, BS; Beaty, TH; Childs, B; Walsh, PC. Family history and the risk of prostate cancer. *Prostate.*, 1990, 17, 337-347.
[8] Ekman, P; Gronberg, H; Matsuyama, H; Kivineva, M; Bergerheim, US; Li, C. Links between genetic and environmental factors and prostate cancer risk. *Prostate.*, 1999, 39, 262-268.
[9] Harlan, LC; Potosky, A; Gilliland, FD; Hoffman, R; Albertsen, PC; Hamilton, AS; Eley, JW; Stanford, JL; Stephenson, RA. Factors associated with initial therapy for clinically localized prostate cancer: prostate cancer outcomes study. *J Natl Cancer Inst.*, 2001, 93, 1864-1871.

[10] Oesterling, JE; Suman, VJ; Zincke, H; Bostwick, DG. PSA-detected (clinical stage T1c or B0) prostate cancer. Pathologically significant tumors. *Urol Clin North Am.*, 1993, 20, 687-693.

[11] Ercole, CJ; Lange, PH; Mathisen, M; Chiou, RK; Reddy, PK; Vessella, RL. Prostatic specific antigen and prostatic acid phosphatase in the monitoring and staging of patients with prostatic cancer. *J Urol.*, 1987, 138, 1181-1184.

[12] Catalona, WJ; Richie, JP; Ahmann, FR; Hudson, MA; Scardino, PT; Flanigan, RC; deKernion, JB; Ratliff, TL; Kavoussi, LR; Dalkin, BL; et al. Comparison of digital rectal examination and serum prostate specific antigen in the early detection of prostate cancer: results of a multicenter clinical trial of 6,630 men. *J Urol.*, 1994, 151, 1283-1290.

[13] Farwell, WR; Linder, JA; Jha, AK. Trends in prostate-specific antigen testing from 1995 through 2004. *Arch Intern Med.*, 2007, 167, 2497-2502.

[14] Andriole, GL; Crawford, ED; Grubb, RL; 3rd; Buys, SS; Chia, D; Church, TR; Fouad, MN; Gelmann, EP; Kvale, PA; Reding, DJ; Weissfeld, JL; Yokochi, LA; O'Brien, B; Clapp, JD; Rathmell, JM; Riley, TL; Hayes, RB; Kramer, BS; Izmirlian, G; Miller, AB; Pinsky, PF; Prorok, PC; Gohagan, JK; Berg, CD. Mortality results from a randomized prostate-cancer screening trial. *N Engl J Med.*, 2009, 360, 1310-1319.

[15] Catalona, WJ; Smith, DS; Ornstein, DK. Prostate cancer detection in men with serum PSA concentrations of 2.6 to 4.0 ng/mL and benign prostate examination. Enhancement of specificity with free PSA measurements. *JAMA.*, 1997, 277, 1452-1455.

[16] Stenman, UH; Leinonen, J; Alfthan, H; Rannikko, S; Tuhkanen, K; Alfthan, O. A complex between prostate-specific antigen and alpha 1-antichymotrypsin is the major form of prostate-specific antigen in serum of patients with prostatic cancer: assay of the complex improves clinical sensitivity for cancer. *Cancer Res.*, 1991, 51, 222-226.

[17] Brawer, MK; Cheli, CD; Neaman, IE; Goldblatt, J; Smith, C; Schwartz, MK; Bruzek, DJ; Morris, DL; Sokoll, LJ; Chan, DW; Yeung, KK; Partin, AW; Allard, WJ. Complexed prostate specific antigen provides significant enhancement of specificity compared with total prostate specific antigen for detecting prostate cancer. *J Urol.*, 2000, 163, 1476-1480.

[18] Benson, MC; Whang, IS; Pantuck, A; Ring, K; Kaplan, SA; Olsson, CA; Cooner, WH. Prostate specific antigen density: a means of

distinguishing benign prostatic hypertrophy and prostate cancer. *J Urol.,* 1992, 147, 815-816.
[19] D'Amico, AV; Renshaw, AA; Sussman, B; Chen, MH. Pretreatment PSA velocity and risk of death from prostate cancer following external beam radiation therapy. *JAMA.,* 2005, 294, 440-447.
[20] Bussemakers, MJ; van Bokhoven, A; Verhaegh, GW; Smit, FP; Karthaus, HF; Schalken, JA; Debruyne, FM; Ru, N; Isaacs, WB. DD3: a new prostate-specific gene, highly overexpressed in prostate cancer. *Cancer Res.,* 1999, 59, 5975-5979.
[21] Horoszewicz, JS; Kawinski, E; Murphy, GP. Monoclonal antibodies to a new antigenic marker in epithelial prostatic cells and serum of prostatic cancer patients. *Anticancer Res,* 1987, 7, 927-935.
[22] Sokoll, LJ; Chan, DW. Prostate-specific antigen. Its discovery and biochemical characteristics. *Urol Clin North Am.,* 1997, 24, 253-259.
[23] Flocks, RH; Urich, VC; Patel, CA; Opitz, JM. Studies on the antigenic properties of prostatic tissue. I. *J Urol.,* 1960, 84, 134-143.
[24] Flocks, RH; Bandhaur, K; Patel, C; Begley, BJ. Studies on spermagglutinating antibodies in antihuman prostate sera. *J Urol.,* 1962, 87, 475-478.
[25] Hara, MIT; Koyanagi, Y; et al. Preparation and immunoelectrophoretic assessment of antisera to human seminal plasma. *Nippon Hoigaku Zasshi.,* 1966, 20.
[26] Ablin, RJ; Soanes, WA; Bronson, P; Witebsky, E. Precipitating antigens of the normal human prostate. *J Reprod Fertil,* 1970, 22, 573-574.
[27] Ablin, RJ. Immunologic studies of normal, benign, and malignant human prostatic tissue. *Cancer.,* 1972, 29, 1570-1574.
[28] Li, TS; Beling, CG. Isolation and characterization of two specific antigens of human seminal plasma. *Fertil Steril,* 1973, 24, 134-144.
[29] Sensabaugh, GF. Isolation and characterization of a semen-specific protein from human seminal plasma: a potential new marker for semen identification. *J Forensic Sci,* 1978, 23, 106-115.
[30] Sensabaugh, GF; Blake, ET. Seminal plasma protein p30: simplified purification and evidence for identity with prostate specific antigen. *J Urol.,* 1990, 144, 1523-1526.
[31] Wang, MC; Valenzuela, LA; Murphy, GP; Chu, TM. Purification of a human prostate specific antigen. *Invest Urol.,* 1979, 17, 159-163.
[32] Wang, MC; Valenzuela, LA; Murphy, GP; Chu, TM. Purification of a human prostate specific antigen. 1979. *J Urol.,* 2002, 167, 960-964; discussion 964-965.

[33] Wang, MC; Valenzuela, LA; Murphy, GP; Chu, TM. Which prostate antigen is which? *Clin Chem.*, 1985, 31, 1405-1406.
[34] Kuriyama, M; Wang, MC; Papsidero, LD; Killian, CS; Shimano, T; Valenzuela, L; Nishiura, T; Murphy, GP; Chu, TM. Quantitation of prostate-specific antigen in serum by a sensitive enzyme immunoassay. *Cancer Res.*, 1980, 40, 4658-4662.
[35] Kuriyama, M; Wang, MC; Lee, CI; Papsidero, LD; Killian, CS; Inaji, H; Slack, NH; Nishiura, T; Murphy, GP; Chu, TM. Use of human prostate-specific antigen in monitoring prostate cancer. *Cancer Res.*, 1981, 41, 3874-3876.
[36] Stamey, TA; Yang, N; Hay, AR; McNeal, JE; Freiha, FS; Redwine, E. Prostate-specific antigen as a serum marker for adenocarcinoma of the prostate. *N Engl J Med.*, 1987, 317, 909-916.
[37] Catalona, WJ; Smith, DS; Ratliff, TL; Dodds, KM; Coplen, DE; Yuan, JJ; Petros, JA; Andriole, GL. Measurement of prostate-specific antigen in serum as a screening test for prostate cancer. *N Engl J Med.*, 1991, 324, 1156-1161.
[38] Kaplan, AP; Silverberg, M. The coagulation-kinin pathway of human plasma. *Blood.*, 1987, 70, 1-15.
[39] Bhoola, KD; Figueroa, CD; Worthy, K. Bioregulation of kinins: kallikreins, kininogens, and kininases. *Pharmacol Rev.*, 1992, 44, 1-80.
[40] Deperthes, D; Marceau, F; Frenette, G; Lazure, C; Tremblay, RR; Dube, JY. Human kallikrein hK2 has low kininogenase activity while prostate-specific antigen (hK3) has none. *Biochim Biophys Acta.*, 1997, 1343, 102-106.
[41] Yousef, GM; Diamandis, EP. The new human tissue kallikrein gene family: structure, function, and association to disease. *Endocr Rev.*, 2001, 22, 184-204.
[42] Yousef, GM; Luo, LY; Diamandis, EP. Identification of novel human kallikrein-like genes on chromosome 19q13.3-q13.4. *Anticancer Res.*, 1999, 19, 2843-2852.
[43] Young, CY; Andrews, PE; Montgomery, BT; Tindall, DJ. Tissue-specific and hormonal regulation of human prostate-specific glandular kallikrein. *Biochemistry.*, 1992, 31, 818-824.
[44] Chapdelaine, P; Paradis, G; Tremblay, RR; Dube, JY. High level of expression in the prostate of a human glandular kallikrein mRNA related to prostate-specific antigen. *FEBS Lett.*, 1988, 236, 205-208.
[45] Henttu, P; Lukkarinen, O; Vihko, P. Expression of the gene coding for human prostate-specific antigen and related hGK-1 in benign and

malignant tumors of the human prostate. *Int J Cancer.,* 1990, 45, 654-660.
[46] Henttu, P; Vihko, P. Prostate-specific antigen and human glandular kallikrein: two kallikreins of the human prostate. *Ann Med.,* 1994, 26, 157-164.
[47] Sinha, AA; Wilson, MJ; Gleason, DF. Immunoelectron microscopic localization of prostatic-specific antigen in human prostate by the protein A-gold complex. *Cancer.,* 1987, 60, 1288-1293.
[48] Frazier, HA; Humphrey, PA; Burchette, JL; Paulson, DF. Immunoreactive prostatic specific antigen in male periurethral glands. *J Urol.,* 1992, 147, 246-248.
[49] Iwakiri, J; Granbois, K; Wehner, N; Graves, HC; Stamey, T. An analysis of urinary prostate specific antigen before and after radical prostatectomy: evidence for secretion of prostate specific antigen by the periurethral glands. *J Urol.,* 1993, 149, 783-786.
[50] Takayama, TK; Vessella, RL; Brawer, MK; True, LD; Noteboom, J; Lange, PH. Urinary prostate specific antigen levels after radical prostatectomy. *J Urol.,* 1994, 151, 82-87.
[51] Lovgren, J; Valtonen-Andre, C; Marsal, K; Lilja, H; Lundwall, A. Measurement of prostate-specific antigen and human glandular kallikrein 2 in different body fluids. *J Androl.,* 1999, 20, 348-355.
[52] Howarth, DJ; Aronson, IB; Diamandis, EP. Immunohistochemical localization of prostate-specific antigen in benign and malignant breast tissues. *Br J Cancer.,* 1997, 75, 1646-1651.
[53] Clements, J; Mukhtar, A. Glandular kallikreins and prostate-specific antigen are expressed in the human endometrium. *J Clin Endocrinol Metab.,* 1994, 78, 1536-1539.
[54] Wang, MC; Papsidero, LD; Kuriyama, M; Valenzuela, LA; Murphy, GP; Chu, TM. Prostate antigen: a new potential marker for prostatic cancer. *Prostate.,* 1981, 2, 89-96.
[55] Chu, TM. Prostate-specific antigen in screening of prostate cancer. *J Clin Lab Anal,* 1994, 8, 323-326.
[56] Riegman, PH; Vlietstra, RJ; van der Korput, HA; Romijn, JC; Trapman, J. Identification and androgen-regulated expression of two major human glandular kallikrein-1 (hGK-1) mRNA species. *Mol Cell Endocrinol.,* 1991, 76, 181-190.
[57] Murtha, P; Tindall, DJ; Young, CY. Androgen induction of a human prostate-specific kallikrein, hKLK2: characterization of an androgen

response element in the 5' promoter region of the gene. *Biochemistry.,* 1993, 32, 6459-6464.

[58] Shan, JD; Porvari, K; Ruokonen, M; Karhu, A; Launonen, V; Hedberg, P; Oikarinen, J; Vihko, P. Steroid-involved transcriptional regulation of human genes encoding prostatic acid phosphatase, prostate-specific antigen, and prostate-specific glandular kallikrein. *Endocrinology.,* 1997, 138, 3764-3770.

[59] Pang, S; Dannull, J; Kaboo, R; Xie, Y; Tso, CL; Michel, K; deKernion, JB; Belldegrun, AS. Identification of a positive regulatory element responsible for tissue-specific expression of prostate-specific antigen. *Cancer Res.,* 1997, 57, 495-499.

[60] Zhang, S; Murtha, PE; Young, CY. Defining a functional androgen responsive element in the 5' far upstream flanking region of the prostate-specific antigen gene. *Biochem Biophys Res Commun.,* 1997, 231, 784-788.

[61] Cleutjens, KB; van der Korput, HA; van Eekelen, CC; van Rooij, HC; Faber, PW; Trapman, J. An androgen response element in a far upstream enhancer region is essential for high, androgen-regulated activity of the prostate-specific antigen promoter. *Mol Endocrinol.,* 1997, 11, 148-161.

[62] clements, J. The molecular biology of the kallikreins and their roles in inflammation. *Farmer SG ed The kinin system , San diego: Academic Press.,* 1997, 72-97.

[63] Lundwall, A; Lilja, H. Molecular cloning of human prostate specific antigen cDNA. *FEBS Lett.,* 1987, 214, 317-322.

[64] Heuze-Vourc'h, N; Leblond, V; Courty, Y. Complex alternative splicing of the hKLK3 gene coding for the tumor marker PSA (prostate-specific-antigen). *Eur J Biochem.,* 2003, 270, 706-714.

[65] Tanaka, T; Isono, T; Yoshiki, T; Yuasa, T; Okada, Y. A novel form of prostate-specific antigen transcript produced by alternative splicing. *Cancer Res.,* 2000, 60, 56-59.

[66] Pampalakis, G; Scorilas, A; Sotiropoulou, G. Novel splice variants of prostate-specific antigen and applications in diagnosis of prostate cancer. *Clin Biochem.,* 2008, 41, 591-597.

[67] Watt, KW; Lee, PJ; M'Timkulu, T; Chan, WP; Loor, R. Human prostate-specific antigen: structural and functional similarity with serine proteases. *Proc Natl Acad Sci U S A.,* 1986, 83, 3166-3170.

[68] Schaller, J; Akiyama, K; Tsuda, R; Hara, M; Marti, T; Rickli, EE. Isolation, characterization and amino-acid sequence of gamma-

seminoprotein, a glycoprotein from human seminal plasma. *Eur J Biochem.*, 1987, 170, 111-120.
[69] Belanger, A; van Halbeek, H; Graves, HC; Grandbois, K; Stamey, TA; Huang, L; Poppe, I; Labrie, F. Molecular mass and carbohydrate structure of prostate specific antigen: studies for establishment of an international PSA standard. *Prostate.*, 1995, 27, 187-197.
[70] Lilja, H. A kallikrein-like serine protease in prostatic fluid cleaves the predominant seminal vesicle protein. *J Clin Invest.*, 1985, 76, 1899-1903.
[71] van Dieijen-Visser, MP; van Pelt, J; Delaere, KP. Pitfalls in the differentiation of N-glycosylation variants of prostate-specific antigen using concanavalin A. *Eur J Clin Chem Clin Biochem.*, 1994, 32, 473-478.
[72] Kumar, A; Mikolajczyk, SD; Goel, AS; Millar, LS; Saedi, MS. Expression of pro form of prostate-specific antigen by mammalian cells and its conversion to mature, active form by human kallikrein 2. *Cancer Res.*, 1997, 57, 3111-3114.
[73] Khan, AR; James, MN. Molecular mechanisms for the conversion of zymogens to active proteolytic enzymes. *Protein Sci.*, 1998, 7, 815-836.
[74] Mikolajczyk, SD; Grauer, LS; Millar, LS; Hill, TM; Kumar, A; Rittenhouse, HG; Wolfert, RL; Saedi, MS. A precursor form of PSA (pPSA) is a component of the free PSA in prostate cancer serum. *Urology.*, 1997, 50, 710-714.
[75] Mikolajczyk, SD; Marker, KM; Millar, LS; Kumar, A; Saedi, MS; Payne, JK; Evans, CL; Gasior, CL; Linton, HJ; Carpenter, P; Rittenhouse, HG. A truncated precursor form of prostate-specific antigen is a more specific serum marker of prostate cancer. *Cancer Res.*, 2001, 61, 6958-6963.
[76] Takayama, TK; Fujikawa, K; Davie, EW. Characterization of the precursor of prostate-specific antigen. Activation by trypsin and by human glandular kallikrein. *J Biol Chem.*, 1997, 272, 21582-21588.
[77] Lovgren, J; Rajakoski, K; Karp, M; Lundwall, a; Lilja, H. Activation of the zymogen form of prostate-specific antigen by human glandular kallikrein 2. *Biochem Biophys Res Commun.*, 1997, 238, 549-555.
[78] Takayama, TK; McMullen, BA; Nelson, PS; Matsumura, M; Fujikawa, K. Characterization of hK4 (prostase), a prostate-specific serine protease: activation of the precursor of prostate specific antigen (pro-PSA) and single-chain urokinase-type plasminogen activator and

degradation of prostatic acid phosphatase. *Biochemistry.*, 2001, 40, 15341-15348.
[79] Villoutreix, BO; Getzoff, ED; Griffin, JH. A structural model for the prostate disease marker, human prostate-specific antigen. *Protein Sci.*, 1994, 3, 2033-2044.
[80] Vihinen, M. Modeling of prostate specific antigen and human glandular kallikrein structures. *Biochem Biophys Res Commun.*, 1994, 204, 1251-1256.
[81] Hassan, MI; Kumar, V; Singh, TP; Yadav, S. Structural model of human PSA: a target for prostate cancer therapy. *Chem Biol Drug Des.*, 2007, 70, 261-267.
[82] Menez, R; Michel, S; Muller, BH; Bossus, M; Ducancel, F; Jolivet-Reynaud, C; Stura, EA. Crystal structure of a ternary complex between humanprostate-specific antigen, its substrate acyl intermediate and an activating antibody. *J Mol Biol.*, 2008, 376, 1021-1033.
[83] Ban, Y; Wang, MC; Watt, KW; Loor, R; Chu, TM. The proteolytic activity of human prostate-specific antigen. *Biochem Biophys Res Commun.*, 1984, 123, 482-488.
[84] Christensson, A; Laurell, CB; Lilja, H. Enzymatic activity of prostate-specific antigen and its reactions with extracellular serine proteinase inhibitors. *Eur J Biochem.*, 1990, 194, 755-763.
[85] Akiyama, K; Nakamura, T; Iwanaga, S; Hara, M. The chymotrypsin-like activity of human prostate-specific antigen, gamma-seminoprotein. *FEBS Lett.*, 1987, 225, 168-172.
[86] Malm, J; Hellman, J; Hogg, P; Lilja, H. Enzymatic action of prostate-specific antigen (PSA or hK3): substrate specificity and regulation by Zn(2+), a tight-binding inhibitor. *Prostate.*, 2000, 45, 132-139.
[87] Christensson, A; Bjork, T; Nilsson, O; Dahlen, U; Matikainen, MT; Cockett, AT; Abrahamsson, PA; Lilja, H. Serum prostate specific antigen complexed to alpha 1-antichymotrypsin as an indicator of prostate cancer. *J Urol.*, 1993, 150, 100-105.
[88] Lilja, H; Christensson, A; Dahlen, U; Matikainen, MT; Nilsson, O; Pettersson, K; Lovgren, T. Prostate-specific antigen in serum occurs predominantly in complex with alpha 1-antichymotrypsin. *Clin Chem.*, 1991, 37, 1618-1625.
[89] Chandra, T; Stackhouse, R; Kidd, VJ; Robson, KJ; Woo, SL. Sequence homology between human alpha 1-antichymotrypsin, alpha 1-antitrypsin, and antithrombin III. *Biochemistry.*, 1983, 22, 5055-5061.

[90] Grauer, LS; Finlay, JA; Mikolajczyk, SD; Pusateri, KD; Wolfert, RL. Detection of human glandular kallikrein, hK2, as its precursor form and in complex with protease inhibitors in prostate carcinoma serum. *J Androl.*, 1998, 19, 407-411.

[91] Rubin, H. The biology and biochemistry of antichymotrypsin and its potential role as a therapeutic agent. *Biol Chem Hoppe Seyler.*, 1992, 373, 497-502.

[92] Clements, JA. The glandular kallikrein family of enzymes: tissue-specific expression and hormonal regulation. *Endocr Rev.*, 1989, 10, 393-419.

[93] Bjartell, A; Bjork, T; Matikainen, MT; Abrahamsson, PA; di Sant'Agnese, A; Lilja, H. Production of alpha-1-antichymotrypsin by PSA-containing cells of human prostate epithelium. *Urology.*, 1993, 42, 502-510.

[94] Song, WWT; Nguyen, C. Western blot and immunohistochemical analysis demonstrates abundant alpha1- antichymotrypsin protein in both peripheral and transition zone prostate tissue in men with normal sized and enlarged prostates. *Journal of Urology.*, 1997, 157, 754.

[95] Christensson, A; Lilja, H. Complex formation between protein C inhibitor and prostate-specific antigen in vitro and in human semen. *Eur J Biochem.*, 1994, 220, 45-53.

[96] Espana, F; Gilabert, J; Estelles, A; Romeu, A; Aznar, J; Cabo, A. Functionally active protein C inhibitor/plasminogen activator inhibitor-3 (PCI/PAI-3) is secreted in seminal vesicles, occurs at high concentrations in human seminal plasma and complexes with prostate-specific antigen. *Thromb Res.*, 1991, 64, 309-320.

[97] Mikolajczyk, SD; Marks, LS; Partin, AW; Rittenhouse, HG. Free prostate-specific antigen in serum is becoming more complex. *Urology.*, 2002, 59, 797-802.

[98] Nurmikko, P; Vaisanen, V; Piironen, T; Lindgren, S; Lilja, H; Pettersson, K. Production and characterization of novel anti-prostate-specific antigen (PSA) monoclonal antibodies that do not detect internally cleaved Lys145-Lys146 inactive PSA. *Clin Chem.*, 2000, 46, 1610-1618.

[99] Mikolajczyk, SD; Millar, LS; Wang, TJ; Rittenhouse, HG; Wolfert, RL; Marks, LS; Song, W; Wheeler, TM; Slawin, KM. "BPSA," a specific molecular form of free prostate-specific antigen, is found predominantly in the transition zone of patients with nodular benign prostatic hyperplasia. *Urology.*, 2000, 55, 41-45.

[100] Mikolajczyk, SD; Millar, LS; Marker, KM; Wang, TJ; Rittenhouse, HG; Marks, LS; Slawin, KM. Seminal plasma contains "BPSA," a molecular form of prostate-specific antigen that is associated with benign prostatic hyperplasia. *Prostate.*, 2000, 45, 271-276.

[101] Linton, HJ; Marks, LS; Millar, LS; Knott, CL; Rittenhouse, HG; Mikolajczyk, SD. Benign prostate-specific antigen (BPSA) in serum is increased in benign prostate disease. *Clin Chem.*, 2003, 49, 253-259.

[102] Mikolajczyk, SD; Millar, LS; Wang, TJ; Rittenhouse, HG; Marks, LS; Song, W; Wheeler, TM; Slawin, KM. A precursor form of prostate-specific antigen is more highly elevated in prostate cancer compared with benign transition zone prostate tissue. *Cancer Res.*, 2000, 60, 756-759.

[103] Steuber, T; Nurmikko, P; Haese, A; Pettersson, K; Graefen, M; Hammerer, P; Huland, H; Lilja, H. Discrimination of benign from malignant prostatic disease by selective measurements of single chain, intact free prostate specific antigen. *J Urol.*, 2002, 168, 1917-1922.

[104] Nurmikko, P; Pettersson, K; Piironen, T; Hugosson, J; Lilja, H. Discrimination of prostate cancer from benign disease by plasma measurement of intact, free prostate-specific antigen lacking an internal cleavage site at Lys145-Lys146. *Clin Chem.*, 2001, 47, 1415-1423.

[105] Sottrup-Jensen, L. Alpha-macroglobulins: structure, shape, and mechanism of proteinase complex formation. *J Biol Chem.*, 1989, 264, 11539-11542.

[106] Catalona, WJ; Hudson, MA; Scardino, PT; Richie, JP; Ahmann, FR; Flanigan, RC; deKernion, JB; Ratliff, TL; Kavoussi, LR; Dalkin, BL; et al. Selection of optimal prostate specific antigen cutoffs for early detection of prostate cancer: receiver operating characteristic curves. *J Urol.*, 1994, 152, 2037-2042.

[107] Sokoloff, RL; WR; Rittenhouse, HG. Standardization of PSA immunoassays: Proposals and practical limitations. *Journal of Clinical Ligand Assay*, 1995, 18, 86-92.

[108] Graves, HC. Issues on standardization of immunoassays for prostate-specific antigen: a review. *Clin Invest Med*, 1993, 16, 415-424.

[109] Nakamura, RM. Current and future directions regarding quality assurance and standardization of prostate specific antigen immunoassays. *Cancer.*, 1994, 74, 1655-1659.

[110] Wu, JT. Assay for prostate specific antigen (PSA): problems and possible solutions. *J Clin Lab Anal*, 1994, 8, 51-62.

[111] Rippey, JH; Wener, MH; Horoszewicz, J; Stenman, UH; Klee, GG; Belanger, A; Maxim, PE; Graves, H; Howanitz, J; Nakamura, RM. Workgroup #1: Standardization of PSA. *Cancer,* 1993, 71, 2678.

[112] Stamey, TA; Prestigiacomo, AF; Chen, Z. Standardization of immunoassays for prostate specific antigen. A different view based on experimental observations. *Cancer,* 1994, 74, 1662-1666.

[113] National Committee for Clinical Laboratory Standards Primary reference preparations used to standardize calibration of immunochemical assays for serum prostate specific antigen (PSA), approved guideline NCCLS Document I/LA19-A ISBN 1-56238-323-X 1997 NCCLS Wayne, PA.

[114] Stamey, TA; Chen, Z; Prestigiacomo, AF. Reference material for PSA: the IFCC standardization study. International Federation of Clinical Chemistry. *Clin Biochem.,* 1998, 31, 475-481.

[115] Rafferty, B; Rigsby, P; Rose, M; Stamey, T; Gaines Das, R. Reference reagents for prostate-specific antigen (PSA): establishment of the first international standards for free PSA and PSA (90:10). *Clin Chem,* 2000, 46, 1310-1317.

[116] Chan, DW; Sokoll, LJ. WHO first international standards for prostate-specific antigen: the beginning of the end for assay discrepancies? *Clin Chem.,* 2000, 46, 1291-1292.

[117] Stephan, C; Kramer, J; Meyer, HA; Kristiansen, G; Ziemer, S; Deger, S; Lein, M; Loening, SA; Jung, K. Different prostate-specific antigen assays give different results on the same blood sample: an obstacle to recommending uniform limits for prostate biopsies. *BJU Int.,* 2007, 99, 1427-1431.

[118] Lilja, H; Oldbring, J; Rannevik, G; Laurell, CB. Seminal vesicle-secreted proteins and their reactions during gelation and liquefaction of human semen. *J Clin Invest.,* 1987, 80, 281-285.

[119] Lilja, H; Abrahamsson, PA; Lundwall, A. Semenogelin, the predominant protein in human semen. Primary structure and identification of closely related proteins in the male accessory sex glands and on the spermatozoa. *J Biol Chem.,* 1989, 264, 1894-1900.

[120] Cohen, P; Graves, HC; Peehl, DM; Kamarei, M; Giudice, LC; Rosenfeld, RG. Prostate-specific antigen (PSA) is an insulin-like growth factor binding protein-3 protease found in seminal plasma. *J Clin Endocrinol Metab.,* 1992, 75, 1046-1053.

[121] Cohen, P; Peehl, DM; Graves, HC; Rosenfeld, RG. Biological effects of prostate specific antigen as an insulin-like growth factor binding protein-3 protease. *J Endocrinol,* 1994, 142, 407-415.
[122] Mantzoros, CS; Tzonou, A; Signorello, LB; Stampfer, M; Trichopoulos, D; Adami, HO. Insulin-like growth factor 1 in relation to prostate cancer and benign prostatic hyperplasia. *Br J Cancer,* 1997, 76, 1115-1118.
[123] Chan, JM; Stampfer, MJ; Giovannucci, E; Gann, PH; Ma, J; Wilkinson, P; Hennekens, CH; Pollak, M. Plasma insulin-like growth factor-I and prostate cancer risk: a prospective study. *Science,* 1998, 279, 563-566.
[124] Kanety, H; Madjar, Y; Dagan, Y; Levi, J; Papa, MZ; Pariente, C; Goldwasser, B; Karasik, A. Serum insulin-like growth factor-binding protein-2 (IGFBP-2) is increased and IGFBP-3 is decreased in patients with prostate cancer: correlation with serum prostate-specific antigen. *J Clin Endocrinol Metab.,* 1993, 77, 229-233.
[125] Niu, Y; Yeh, S; Miyamoto, H; Li, G; Altuwaijri, S; Yuan, J; Han, R; Ma, T; Kuo, HC; Chang, C. Tissue prostate-specific antigen facilitates refractory prostate tumor progression via enhancing ARA70-regulated androgen receptor transactivation. *Cancer Res,* 2008, 68, 7110-7119.
[126] Killian, CS; Corral, DA; Kawinski, E; Constantine, RI. Mitogenic response of osteoblast cells to prostate-specific antigen suggests an activation of latent TGF-beta and a proteolytic modulation of cell adhesion receptors. *Biochem Biophys Res Commun.,* 1993, 192, 940-947.
[127] Cramer, SD; Chen, Z; Peehl, DM. Prostate specific antigen cleaves parathyroid hormone-related protein in the PTH-like domain: inactivation of PTHrP-stimulated cAMP accumulation in mouse osteoblasts. *J Urol.,* 1996, 156, 526-531.
[128] Iwamura, M; Hellman, J; Cockett, AT; Lilja, H; Gershagen, S. Alteration of the hormonal bioactivity of parathyroid hormone-related protein (PTHrP) as a result of limited proteolysis by prostate-specific antigen. *Urology.,* 1996, 48, 317-325.
[129] Mattsson, JM; Laakkonen, P; Stenman, UH; Koistinen, H. Antiangiogenic properties of prostate-specific antigen (PSA). *Scand J Clin Lab Invest.,* 2009, 69, 447-451.
[130] Yu, H; Diamandis, EP; Zarghami, N; Grass, L. Induction of prostate specific antigen production by steroids and tamoxifen in breast cancer cell lines. *Breast Cancer Res Treat.,* 1994, 32, 291-300.

[131] Monne, M; Croce, CM; Yu, H; Diamandis, EP. Molecular characterization of prostate-specific antigen messenger RNA expressed in breast tumors. *Cancer Res.,* 1994, 54, 6344-6347.

[132] Yu, H; Giai, M; Diamandis, EP; Katsaros, D; Sutherland, DJ; Levesque, MA; Roagna, R; Ponzone, R; Sismondi, P. Prostate-specific antigen is a new favorable prognostic indicator for women with breast cancer. *Cancer Res.,* 1995, 55, 2104-2110.

[133] Denmeade, SR; Nagy, A; Gao, J; Lilja, H; Schally, AV; Isaacs, JT. Enzymatic activation of a doxorubicin-peptide prodrug by prostate-specific antigen. *Cancer Res,* 1998, 58, 2537-2540.

[134] Khan, SR; Denmeade, SR. In vivo activity of a PSA-activated doxorubicin prodrug against PSA-producing human prostate cancer xenografts. *Prostate.,* 2000, 45, 80-83.

[135] Tombal, B; Weeraratna, AT; Denmeade, SR; Isaacs, JT. Thapsigargin induces a calmodulin/calcineurin-dependent apoptotic cascade responsible for the death of prostatic cancer cells. *Prostate.,* 2000, 43, 303-317.

[136] Papsidero, LD; Wang, MC; Valenzuela, LA; Murphy, GP; Chu, TM. A prostate antigen in sera of prostatic cancer patients. *Cancer Res.,* 1980, 40, 2428-2432.

[137] Wang, TJ; Rittenhouse, HG; Wolfert, RL; Lynne, CM; Brackett, NL. PSA concentrations in seminal plasma. *Clin Chem.,* 1998, 44, 895-896.

[138] Klein, LT; Lowe, FC. The effects of prostatic manipulation on prostate-specific antigen levels. *Urol Clin North Am.,* 1997, 24, 293-297.

[139] Rana, A; Chisholm, GD. He sold his bike for a low prostate specific antigen. *J Urol.,* 1994, 151, 700.

[140] Oremek, GM; Seiffert, UB. Physical activity releases prostate-specific antigen (PSA) from the prostate gland into blood and increases serum PSA concentrations. *Clin Chem.,* 1996, 42, 691-695.

[141] Tchetgen, MB; Song, JT; Strawderman, M; Jacobsen, SJ; Oesterling, JE. Ejaculation increases the serum prostate-specific antigen concentration. *Urology.,* 1996, 47, 511-516.

[142] Herschman, JD; Smith, DS; Catalona, WJ. Effect of ejaculation on serum total and free prostate-specific antigen concentrations. *Urology.,* 1997, 50, 239-243.

[143] Guess, HA; Heyse, JF; Gormley, GJ. The effect of finasteride on prostate-specific antigen in men with benign prostatic hyperplasia. *Prostate.,* 1993, 22, 31-37.

[144] Roehrborn, CG; Boyle, P; Nickel, JC; Hoefner, K; Andriole, G. Efficacy and safety of a dual inhibitor of 5-alpha-reductase types 1 and 2 (dutasteride) in men with benign prostatic hyperplasia. *Urology.,* 2002, 60, 434-441.

[145] Vieira, JG; Nishida, SK; Pereira, AB; Arraes, RF; Verreschi, IT. Serum levels of prostate-specific antigen in normal boys throughout puberty. *J Clin Endocrinol Metab,* 1994, 78, 1185-1187.

[146] Oesterling, JE; Cooner, WH; Jacobsen, SJ; Guess, HA; Lieber, MM. Influence of patient age on the serum PSA concentration. An important clinical observation. *Urol Clin North Am,* 1993, 20, 671-680.

[147] Hankey, BF; Feuer, EJ; Clegg, LX; Hayes, RB; Legler, JM; Prorok, PC; Ries, LA; Merrill, RM; Kaplan, RS. Cancer surveillance series: interpreting trends in prostate cancer--part I: Evidence of the effects of screening in recent prostate cancer incidence, mortality, and survival rates. *J Natl Cancer Inst.,* 1999, 91, 1017-1024.

[148] Chu, KC; Tarone, RE; Freeman, HP. Trends in prostate cancer mortality among black men and white men in the United States. *Cancer.,* 2003, 97, 1507-1516.

[149] Schroder, FH; van der Maas, P; Beemsterboer, P; Kruger, AB; Hoedemaeker, R; Rietbergen, J; Kranse, R. Evaluation of the digital rectal examination as a screening test for prostate cancer. Rotterdam section of the European Randomized Study of Screening for Prostate Cancer. *J Natl Cancer Inst.,* 1998, 90, 1817-1823.

[150] Littrup, PJ; Kane, RA; Mettlin, CJ; Murphy, GP; Lee, F; Toi, A; Badalament, R; Babaian, R. Cost-effective prostate cancer detection. Reduction of low-yield biopsies. Investigators of the American Cancer Society National Prostate Cancer Detection Project. *Cancer.,* 1994, 74, 3146-3158.

[151] Andriole, GL; Levin, DL; Crawford, ED; Gelmann, EP; Pinsky, PF; Chia, D; Kramer, BS; Reding, D; Church, TR; Grubb, RL; Izmirlian, G; Ragard, LR; Clapp, JD; Prorok, PC; Gohagan, JK. Prostate Cancer Screening in the Prostate, Lung, Colorectal and Ovarian (PLCO) Cancer Screening Trial: findings from the initial screening round of a randomized trial. *J Natl Cancer Inst,* 2005, 97, 433-438.

[152] Catalona, WJ; Partin, AW; Slawin, KM; Brawer, MK; Flanigan, RC; Patel, A; Richie, JP; deKernion, JB; Walsh, PC; Scardino, PT; Lange, PH; Subong, EN; Parson, RE; Gasior, GH; Loveland, KG; Southwick, PC. Use of the percentage of free prostate-specific antigen to enhance

differentiation of prostate cancer from benign prostatic disease: a prospective multicenter clinical trial. *JAMA,* 1998, 279, 1542-1547.

[153] Stenman, UH; Hakama, M; Knekt, P; Aromaa, A; Teppo, L; Leinonen, J. Serum concentrations of prostate specific antigen and its complex with alpha 1-antichymotrypsin before diagnosis of prostate cancer. *Lancet.,* 1994, 344, 1594-1598.

[154] Lilja, H; Ulmert, D; Bjork, T; Becker, C; Serio, AM; Nilsson, JA; Abrahamsson, PA; Vickers, AJ; Berglund, G. Long-term prediction of prostate cancer up to 25 years before diagnosis of prostate cancer using prostate kallikreins measured at age 44 to 50 years. *J Clin Oncol,* 2007, 25, 431-436.

[155] Ulmert, D; Cronin, AM; Bjork, T; O'Brien, MF; Scardino, PT; Eastham, JA; Becker, C; Berglund, G; Vickers, AJ; Lilja, H. Prostate-specific antigen at or before age 50 as a predictor of advanced prostate cancer diagnosed up to 25 years later: a case-control study. *BMC Med.,* 2008, 6, 6.

[156] Vickers, AJ; Ulmert, D; Serio, AM; Bjork, T; Scardino, PT; Eastham, JA; Berglund, G; Lilja, H. The predictive value of prostate cancer biomarkers depends on age and time to diagnosis: towards a biologically-based screening strategy. *Int J Cancer,* 2007, 121, 2212-2217.

[157] Gann, PH; Hennekens, CH; Stampfer, MJ. A prospective evaluation of plasma prostate-specific antigen for detection of prostatic cancer. *JAMA.,* 1995, 273, 289-294.

[158] Antenor, JA; Han, M; Roehl, KA; Nadler, RB; Catalona, WJ. Relationship between initial prostate specific antigen level and subsequent prostate cancer detection in a longitudinal screening study. *J Urol,* 2004, 172, 90-93.

[159] Crawford, ED; DeAntoni, EP; Etzioni, R; Schaefer, VC; Olson, RM; Ross, CA. Serum prostate-specific antigen and digital rectal examination for early detection of prostate cancer in a national community-based program. The Prostate Cancer Education Council. *Urology,* 1996, 47, 863-869.

[160] Hugosson, J; Aus, G; Lilja, H; Lodding, P; Pihl, CG. Results of a randomized, population-based study of biennial screening using serum prostate-specific antigen measurement to detect prostate carcinoma. *Cancer,* 2004, 100, 1397-1405.

[161] Leinonen, J; Lovgren, T; Vornanen, T; Stenman, UH. Double-label time-resolved immunofluorometric assay of prostate-specific antigen

and of its complex with alpha 1-antichymotrypsin. *Clin Chem.*, 1993, 39, 2098-2103.

[162] Lilja, H. Significance of different molecular forms of serum PSA. The free, noncomplexed form of PSA versus that complexed to alpha 1-antichymotrypsin. *Urol Clin North Am.*, 1993, 20, 681-686.

[163] Luderer, AA; Chen, YT; Soriano, TF; Kramp, WJ; Carlson, G; Cuny, C; Sharp, T; Smith, W; Petteway, J; Brawer, MK; et al. Measurement of the proportion of free to total prostate-specific antigen improves diagnostic performance of prostate-specific antigen in the diagnostic gray zone of total prostate-specific antigen. *Urology,* 1995, 46, 187-194.

[164] Catalona, WJ; Smith, DS; Wolfert, RL; Wang, TJ; Rittenhouse, HG; Ratliff, TL; Nadler, RB. Evaluation of percentage of free serum prostate-specific antigen to improve specificity of prostate cancer screening. *JAMA,* 1995, 274, 1214-1220.

[165] Bangma, CH; Kranse, R; Blijenberg, BG; Schroder, FH. The value of screening tests in the detection of prostate cancer. Part I: Results of a retrospective evaluation of 1726 men. *Urology* 1995, 46, 773-778.

[166] Bangma, CH; Kranse, R; Blijenberg, BG; Schroder, FH. The value of screening tests in the detection of prostate cancer. Part II: Retrospective analysis of free/total prostate-specific analysis ratio, age-specific reference ranges, and PSA density. *Urology* 1995, 46, 779-784.

[167] Peter, J; Unverzagt, C; Krogh, TN; Vorm, O; Hoesel, W. Identification of precursor forms of free prostate-specific antigen in serum of prostate cancer patients by immunosorption and mass spectrometry. *Cancer Res,* 2001, 61, 957-962.

[168] Brawer, MK. Clinical usefulness of assays for complexed prostate-specific antigen. *Urol Clin North Am,* 2002, 29, 193-203, xi.

[169] Partin, AW; Brawer, MK; Bartsch, G; Horninger, W; Taneja, SS; Lepor, H; Babaian, R; Childs, SJ; Stamey, T; Fritsche, HA; Sokoll, L; Chan, DW; Thiel, RP; Cheli, CD. Complexed prostate specific antigen improves specificity for prostate cancer detection: results of a prospective multicenter clinical trial. *J Urol,* 2003, 170, 1787-1791.

[170] Okegawa, T; Noda, H; Nutahara, K; Higashihara, E. Comparison of two investigative assays for the complexed prostate-specific antigen in total prostate-specific antigen between 4.1 and 10.0 ng/mL. *Urology,* 2000, 55, 700-704.

[171] Parsons, JK; Brawer, MK; Cheli, CD; Partin, AW; Djavan, R. Complexed prostate specific antigen (PSA) reduces unnecessary prostate

biopsies in the 2.6-4.0 ng/mL range of total PSA. *BJU Int,* 2004, 94, 47-50.

[172] Carter, HB; Pearson, JD; Metter, EJ; Brant, LJ; Chan, DW; Andres, R; Fozard, JL; Walsh, PC. Longitudinal evaluation of prostate-specific antigen levels in men with and without prostate disease. *JAMA,* 1992, 267, 2215-2220.

[173] Partin, AW; Carter, HB; Chan, DW; Epstein, JI; Oesterling, JE; Rock, RC; Weber, JP; Walsh, PC. Prostate specific antigen in the staging of localized prostate cancer: influence of tumor differentiation, tumor volume and benign hyperplasia. *J Urol,* 1990, 143, 747-752.

[174] Meyer, JS; Sufrin, G; Martin, SA. Proliferative activity of benign human prostate, prostatic adenocarcinoma and seminal vesicle evaluated by thymidine labeling. *J Urol,* 1982, 128, 1353-1356.

[175] Mettlin, C; Littrup, PJ; Kane, RA; Murphy, GP; Lee, F; Chesley, A; Badalament, R; Mostofi, FK. Relative sensitivity and specificity of serum prostate specific antigen (PSA) level compared with age-referenced PSA, PSA density, and PSA change. Data from the American Cancer Society National Prostate Cancer Detection Project. *Cancer* 1994, 74, 1615-1620.

[176] Smith, DS; Catalona, WJ. Rate of change in serum prostate specific antigen levels as a method for prostate cancer detection. *J Urol,* 1994, 152, 1163-1167.

[177] Carter, HB; Pearson, JD. Prostate-specific antigen velocity and repeated measures of prostate-specific antigen. *Urol Clin North Am,* 1997, 24, 333-338.

[178] Prestigiacomo, AF; Stamey, TA. Physiological variation of serum prostate specific antigen in the 4.0 to 10.0 ng./ml. range in male volunteers. *J Urol* 1996, 155, 1977-1980.

[179] Kadmon, D; Weinberg, AD; Williams, RH; Pavlik, VN; Cooper, P; Migliore, PJ. Pitfalls in interpreting prostate specific antigen velocity. *J Urol,* 1996, 155, 1655-1657.

[180] Komatsu, K; Wehner, N; Prestigiacomo, AF; Chen, Z; Stamey, TA. Physiologic (intraindividual) variation of serum prostate-specific antigen in 814 men from a screening population. *Urology,* 1996, 47, 343-346.

[181] Yuan, JJ; Coplen, DE; Petros, JA; Figenshau, RS; Ratliff, TL; Smith, DS; Catalona, WJ. Effects of rectal examination, prostatic massage, ultrasonography and needle biopsy on serum prostate specific antigen levels. *J Urol,* 1992, 147, 810-814.

[182] Carter, HB; Pearson, JD; Waclawiw, Z; Metter, EJ; Chan, DW; Guess, HA; Walsh, PC. Prostate-specific antigen variability in men without prostate cancer: effect of sampling interval on prostate-specific antigen velocity. *Urology,* 1995, 45, 591-596.

[183] Fang, J; Metter, EJ; Landis, P; Carter, HB. PSA velocity for assessing prostate cancer risk in men with PSA levels between 2.0 and 4.0 ng/ml. *Urology,* 2002, 59, 889-893, discussion 893-884.

[184] Vickers, AJ; Savage, C; O'Brien, MF; Lilja, H. Systematic review of pretreatment prostate-specific antigen velocity and doubling time as predictors for prostate cancer. *J Clin Oncol,* 2009, 27, 398-403.

[185] Benson, MC; Whang, IS; Olsson, CA; McMahon, DJ; Cooner, WH. The use of prostate specific antigen density to enhance the predictive value of intermediate levels of serum prostate specific antigen. *J Urol,* 1992, 147, 817-821.

[186] Rommel, FM; Agusta, VE; Breslin, JA; Huffnagle, HW; Pohl, CE; Sieber, PR; Stahl, CA. The use of prostate specific antigen and prostate specific antigen density in the diagnosis of prostate cancer in a community based urology practice. *J Urol* 1994, 151, 88-93.

[187] Seaman, E; Whang, M; Olsson, CA; Katz, A; Cooner, WH; Benson, MC. PSA density (PSAD). Role in patient evaluation and management. *Urol Clin North Am,* 1993, 20, 653-663.

[188] Bazinet, M; Meshref, AW; Trudel, C; Aronson, S; Peloquin, F; Nachabe, M; Begin, LR; Elhilali, MM. Prospective evaluation of prostate-specific antigen density and systematic biopsies for early detection of prostatic carcinoma. *Urology.,* 1994, 43, 44-51, discussion 51-42.

[189] Lujan, M; Paez, A; Llanes, L; Miravalles, E; Berenguer, A. Prostate specific antigen density. Is there a role for this parameter when screening for prostate cancer? *Prostate Cancer Prostatic Dis,* 2001, 4, 146-149.

[190] Uzzo RG; Wei JT; Waldbaum RS; Perlmutter AP; Byrne JC; Vaughan ED; Jr. The influence of prostate size on cancer detection. *Urology* 1995, 46, 831-836.

[191] Taneja, SS; Tran, K; Lepor, H. Volume-specific cutoffs are necessary for reproducible application of prostate-specific antigen density of the transition zone in prostate cancer detection. *Urology.,* 2001, 58, 222-227.

[192] Cooner, WH. Prostate cancer. *J Urol,* 1994, 151, 103-104.

[193] Keetch, DW; McMurtry, JM; Smith, DS; Andriole, GL; Catalona, WJ. Prostate specific antigen density versus prostate specific antigen slope as

predictors of prostate cancer in men with initially negative prostatic biopsies. *J Urol,* 1996, 156, 428-431.
[194] Catalona, WJ; Southwick, PC; Slawin, KM; Partin, AW; Brawer, MK; Flanigan, RC; Patel, A; Richie, JP; Walsh, PC; Scardino, PT; Lange, PH; Gasior, GH; Loveland, KG; Bray, KR. Comparison of percent free PSA, PSA density, and age-specific PSA cutoffs for prostate cancer detection and staging. *Urology,* 2000, 56, 255-260.
[195] Oesterling, JE; Jacobsen, SJ; Chute, CG; Guess, HA; Girman, CJ; Panser, LA; Lieber, MM. Serum prostate-specific antigen in a community-based population of healthy men. Establishment of age-specific reference ranges. *JAMA,* 1993, 270, 860-864.
[196] Morgan, TO; Jacobsen, SJ; McCarthy, WF; Jacobson, DJ; McLeod, DG; Moul, JW. Age-specific reference ranges for prostate-specific antigen in black men. *N Engl J Med,* 1996, 335, 304-310.
[197] Crawford, ED; Leewansangtong, S; Goktas, S; Holthaus, K; Baier, M. Efficiency of prostate-specific antigen and digital rectal examination in screening, using 4.0 ng/ml and age-specific reference range as a cutoff for abnormal values. *Prostate,* 1999, 38, 296-302.
[198] Thompson, IM; Ankerst, DP; Chi, C; Lucia, MS; Goodman, PJ; Crowley, JJ; Parnes, HL; Coltman, CA. Jr. Operating characteristics of prostate-specific antigen in men with an initial PSA level of 3.0 ng/ml or lower. *JAMA,* 2005, 294, 66-70.
[199] Thompson, IM; Pauler, DK; Goodman, PJ; Tangen, CM; Lucia, MS; Parnes, HL; Minasian, LM; Ford, LG; Lippman, SM; Crawford, ED; Crowley, JJ; Coltman, CA. Jr. Prevalence of prostate cancer among men with a prostate-specific antigen level < or =4.0 ng per milliliter. *N Engl J Med,* 2004, 350, 2239-2246.
[200] Piironen, T; Lovgren, J; Karp, M; Eerola, R; Lundwall, A; Dowell, B; Lovgren, T; Lilja, H; Pettersson, K. Immunofluorometric assay for sensitive and specific measurement of human prostatic glandular kallikrein (hK2) in serum. *Clin Chem,* 1996, 42, 1034-1041.
[201] Finlay, JA; Evans, CL; Day, JR; Payne, JK; Mikolajczyk, SD; Millar, LS; Kuus-Reichel, K; Wolfert, RL; Rittenhouse, HG. Development of monoclonal antibodies specific for human glandular kallikrein (hK2): development of a dual antibody immunoassay for hK2 with negligible prostate-specific antigen cross-reactivity. *Urology,* 1998, 51, 804-809.
[202] Darson, MF; Pacelli, A; Roche, P; Rittenhouse, HG; Wolfert, RL; Young, CY; Klee, GG; Tindall, DJ; Bostwick, DG. Human glandular kallikrein 2 (hK2) expression in prostatic intraepithelial neoplasia and

adenocarcinoma: a novel prostate cancer marker. *Urology,* 1997, 49, 857-862.
[203] Darson, MF; Pacelli, A; Roche, P; Rittenhouse, HG; Wolfert, RL; Saeid, MS; Young, CY; Klee, GG; Tindall, DJ; Bostwick, DG. Human glandular kallikrein 2 expression in prostate adenocarcinoma and lymph node metastases. *Urology,* 1999, 53, 939-944.
[204] Tremblay, RR; Deperthes, D; Tetu, B; Dube, JY. Immunohistochemical study suggesting a complementary role of kallikreins hK2 and hK3 (prostate-specific antigen) in the functional analysis of human prostate tumors. *Am J Pathol,* 1997, 150, 455-459.
[205] Partin, AW; Catalona, WJ; Finlay, JA; Darte, C; Tindall, DJ; Young, CY; Klee, GG; Chan, DW; Rittenhouse, HG; Wolfert, RL; Woodrum DL. Use of human glandular kallikrein 2 for the detection of prostate cancer: preliminary analysis. *Urology,* 1999, 54, 839-845.
[206] Becker, C; Piironen, T; Kiviniemi, J; Lilja, H; Pettersson, K. Sensitive and specific immunodetection of human glandular kallikrein 2 in serum. *Clin Chem,* 2000, 46, 198-206.
[207] Haese, A; Becker, C; Noldus, J; Graefen, M; Huland, E; Huland, H; Lilja, H. Human glandular kallikrein 2: a potential serum marker for predicting the organ confined versus non-organ confined growth of prostate cancer. *J Urol,* 2000, 163, 1491-1497.
[208] Nam, RK; Diamandis, EP; Toi, A; Trachtenberg, J; Magklara, A; Scorilas, A; Papnastasiou, PA; Jewett, MA; Narod, SA. Serum human glandular kallikrein-2 protease levels predict the presence of prostate cancer among men with elevated prostate-specific antigen. *J Clin Oncol,* 2000, 18, 1036-1042.
[209] Xi, Z; Klokk, TI; Korkmaz, K; Kurys, P; Elbi, C; Risberg, B; Danielsen, H; Loda, M; Saatcioglu, F. Kallikrein 4 is a predominantly nuclear protein and is overexpressed in prostate cancer. *Cancer Res.,* 2004, 64, 2365-2370.
[210] Stephan, C; Meyer, HA; Cammann, H; Nakamura, T; Diamandis, EP; Jung, K. Improved prostate cancer detection with a human kallikrein 11 and percentage free PSA-based artificial neural network. *Biol Chem.,* 2006, 387, 801-805.
[211] Hooper, JD; Bui, LT; Rae, FK; Harvey, TJ; Myers, SA; Ashworth, LK; Clements, JA. Identification and characterization of KLK14, a novel kallikrein serine protease gene located on human chromosome 19q13.4 and expressed in prostate and skeletal muscle. *Genomics.,* 2001, 73, 117-122.

[212] Stephan, C; Yousef, GM; Scorilas, A; Jung, K; Jung, M; Kristiansen, G; Hauptmann, S; Bharaj, BS; Nakamura, T; Loening, SA; Diamandis, EP. Quantitative analysis of kallikrein 15 gene expression in prostate tissue. *J Urol.,* 2003, 169, 361-364.

[213] Fair, WR; Israeli, RS; Heston, WD. Prostate-specific membrane antigen. *Prostate.,* 1997, 32, 140-148.

[214] Israeli, RS; Grob, M; Fair, WR. Prostate-specific membrane antigen and other prostatic tumor markers on the horizon. *Urol Clin North Am,* 1997, 24, 439-450.

[215] Bostwick, DG; Pacelli, A; Blute, M; Roche, P; Murphy, GP. Prostate specific membrane antigen expression in prostatic intraepithelial neoplasia and adenocarcinoma: a study of 184 cases. *Cancer,* 1998, 82, 2256-2261.

[216] Sweat, SD; Pacelli, A; Murphy, GP; Bostwick, DG. Prostate-specific membrane antigen expression is greatest in prostate adenocarcinoma and lymph node metastases. *Urology,* 1998, 52, 637-640.

[217] Murphy, GP; Holmes, EH; Boynton, AL; Kenny, GM; Ostenson, RC; Erickson, SJ; Barren, RJ. Comparison of prostate specific antigen, prostate specific membrane antigen, and LNCaP-based enzyme-linked immunosorbent assays in prostatic cancer patients and patients with benign prostatic enlargement. *Prostate,* 1995, 26, 164-168.

[218] Rochon, YP; Horoszewicz, JS; Boynton, AL; Holmes, EH; Barren, RJ; 3rd; Erickson, SJ; Kenny, GM; Murphy, GP. Western blot assay for prostate-specific membrane antigen in serum of prostate cancer patients. *Prostate,* 1994, 25, 219-223.

[219] Murphy, GP. Radioscintiscanning of prostate cancer. *Cancer,* 2006, 75, 1819-1822.

[220] Elgamal, AA; Holmes, EH; Su, SL; Tino, WT; Simmons, SJ; Peterson, M; Greene, TG; Boynton, AL; Murphy, GP. Prostate-specific membrane antigen (PSMA): current benefits and future value. *Semin Surg Oncol,* 2000, 18, 10-16.

[221] Schalken, JA; Hessels, D; Verhaegh, G. New targets for therapy in prostate cancer: differential display code 3 (DD3(PCA3)), a highly prostate cancer-specific gene. *Urology,* 2003, 62, 34-43.

[222] de Kok JB; Verhaegh GW; Roelofs RW; Hessels D; Kiemeney LA; Aalders TW; Swinkels DW; Schalken JA. DD3(PCA3), a very sensitive and specific marker to detect prostate tumors. *Cancer Res,* 2002, 62, 2695-2698.

[223] Landers, KA; Burger, MJ; Tebay, MA; Purdie, DM; Scells, B; Samaratunga, H; Lavin, MF; Gardiner, RA. Use of multiple biomarkers for a molecular diagnosis of prostate cancer. *Int J Cancer,* 2005, 114, 950-956.

[224] van Gils, MP; Cornel, EB; Hessels, D; Peelen, WP; Witjes, JA; Mulders, PF; Rittenhouse, HG; Schalken, JA. Molecular PCA3 diagnostics on prostatic fluid. *Prostate.,* 2007, 67, 881-887.

[225] Groskopf, J; Aubin, SM; Deras, IL; Blase, A; Bodrug, S; Clark, C; Brentano, S; Mathis, J; Pham, J; Meyer, T; Cass, M; Hodge, P; Macairan, ML; Marks, LS; Rittenhouse, H. APTIMA PCA3 molecular urine test: development of a method to aid in the diagnosis of prostate cancer. *Clin Chem.,* 2006, 52, 1089-1095.

[226] van Gils, MP; Hessels, D; van Hooij, O; Jannink, SA; Peelen, WP; Hanssen, SL; Witjes, JA; Cornel, EB; Karthaus, HF; Smits, GA; Dijkman, GA; Mulders, PF; Schalken, JA. The time-resolved fluorescence-based PCA3 test on urinary sediments after digital rectal examination, a Dutch multicenter validation of the diagnostic performance. *Clin Cancer Res.,* 2007, 13, 939-943.

[227] Tinzl, M; Marberger, M; Horvath, S; Chypre, C. DD3PCA3 RNA analysis in urine--a new perspective for detecting prostate cancer. *Eur Urol.,* 2004, 46, 182-186, discussion 187.

[228] Sardana, G; Dowell, B; Diamandis, EP. Emerging biomarkers for the diagnosis and prognosis of prostate cancer. *Clin Chem.,* 2008, 54, 1951-1960.

[229] Bensalah, K; Lotan, Y; Karam, JA; Shariat, SF. New circulating biomarkers for prostate cancer. *Prostate Cancer Prostatic Dis.,* 2008, 11, 112-120.

[230] Amling, CL; Bergstralh, EJ; Blute, ML; Slezak, JM; Zincke, H. Defining prostate specific antigen progression after radical prostatectomy: what is the most appropriate cut point? *J Urol,* 2001, 165, 1146-1151.

[231] Freedland, SJ; Sutter, ME; Dorey, F; Aronson, WJ. Defining the ideal cutpoint for determining PSA recurrence after radical prostatectomy. Prostate-specific antigen. *Urology.,* 2003, 61, 365-369.

[232] Pound, CR; Partin, AW; Epstein, JI; Walsh, PC. Prostate-specific antigen after anatomic radical retropubic prostatectomy. Patterns of recurrence and cancer control. *Urol Clin North Am.,* 1997, 24, 395-406.

[233] Partin, AW; Pearson, JD; Landis, PK; Carter, HB; Pound, CR; Clemens, JQ; Epstein, JI; Walsh, PC. Evaluation of serum prostate-specific

antigen velocity after radical prostatectomy to distinguish local recurrence from distant metastases. *Urology* 1994, 43, 649-659.

[234] Horwitz, EM; Thames, HD; Kuban, DA; Levy, LB; Kupelian, PA; Martinez, AA; Michalski, JM; Pisansky, TM; Sandler, HM; Shipley, WU; Zelefsky, MJ; Hanks, GE; Zietman, AL. Definitions of biochemical failure that best predict clinical failure in patients with prostate cancer treated with external beam radiation alone: a multi-institutional pooled analysis. *J Urol.,* 2005, 173, 797-802.

[235] Pound, CR; Partin, AW; Eisenberger, MA; Chan, DW; Pearson, JD; Walsh, PC. Natural history of progression after PSA elevation following radical prostatectomy. *JAMA,* 1999, 281, 1591-1597.

[236] Freedland, SJ; Humphreys, EB; Mangold, LA; Eisenberger, M; Dorey, FJ; Walsh, PC; Partin, AW. Risk of prostate cancer-specific mortality following biochemical recurrence after radical prostatectomy. *JAMA,* 2005, 294, 433-439.

[237] Epstein, JI; Pizov, G; Walsh, PC. Correlation of pathologic findings with progression after radical retropubic prostatectomy. *Cancer,* 1993, 71, 3582-3593.

[238] Norberg, M; Holmberg, L; Wheeler, T; Magnusson, A. Five year follow-up after radical prostatectomy for localized prostate cancer--a study of the impact of different tumor variables on progression. *Scand J Urol Nephrol,* 1994, 28, 391-399.

[239] Ravery, V; Boccon-Gibod, LA; Meulemans, A; Dauge-Geffroy, MC; Toublanc, M; Boccon-Gibod, L. Predictive value of pathological features for progression after radical prostatectomy. *Eur Urol,* 1994, 26, 197-201.

[240] Partin, AW; Piantadosi, S; Sanda, MG; Epstein, JI; Marshall, FF; Mohler, JL; Brendler CB; Walsh, PC; Simons, JW. Selection of men at high risk for disease recurrence for experimental adjuvant therapy following radical prostatectomy. *Urology,* 1995, 45, 831-838.

[241] Lerner, SE; Blute, ML; Bergstralh, EJ; Bostwick, DG; Eickholt, JT; Zincke, H. Analysis of risk factors for progression in patients with pathologically confined prostate cancers after radical retropubic prostatectomy. *J Urol,* 1996, 156, 137-143.

[242] Bauer, JJ; Sesterhenn, IA; Mostofi, FK; McLeod, DG; Srivastava, S; Moul, JW. Elevated levels of apoptosis regulator proteins p53 and bcl-2 are independent prognostic biomarkers in surgically treated clinically localized prostate cancer. *J Urol,* 1996, 156, 1511-1516.

[243] Bettencourt, MC; Bauer, JJ; Sesterhenn, IA; Mostofi, FK; McLeod, DG; Moul, JW. Ki-67 expression is a prognostic marker of prostate cancer recurrence after radical prostatectomy. *J Urol,* 1996, 156, 1064-1068.
[244] Bauer, JJ; Connelly, RR; Sesterhenn, IA; Bettencourt, MC; McLeod, DG; Srivastava, S; Moul, JW. Biostatistical modeling using traditional variables and genetic biomarkers for predicting the risk of prostate carcinoma recurrence after radical prostatectomy. *Cancer.,* 1997, 79, 952-962.
[245] Isaacs, JT. Molecular markers for prostate cancer metastasis. Developing diagnostic methods for predicting the aggressiveness of prostate cancer. *Am J Pathol,* 1997, 150, 1511-1521.
[246] Bostwick, DG. Practical clinical application of predictive factors in prostate cancer. A review with an emphasis on quantitative methods in tissue specimens. *Anal Quant Cytol Histol,* 1998, 20, 323-342.
[247] Moul, JW; Connelly, RR; Perahia, B; McLeod, DG. The contemporary value of pretreatment prostatic acid phosphatase to predict pathological stage and recurrence in radical prostatectomy cases. *J Urol,* 1998, 159, 935-940.
[248] Cordon-Cardo, C; Koff, A; Drobnjak, M; Capodieci, P; Osman, I; Millard, SS; Gaudin, PB; Fazzari, M; Zhang, ZF; Massague, J; Scher, HI. Distinct altered patterns of p27KIP1 gene expression in benign prostatic hyperplasia and prostatic carcinoma. *J Natl Cancer Inst.,* 1998, 90, 1284-1291.
[249] Kattan, MW; Eastham, JA; Stapleton, AM; Wheeler, TM; Scardino, PT. A preoperative nomogram for disease recurrence following radical prostatectomy for prostate cancer. *J Natl Cancer Inst.,* 1998, 90, 766-771.
[250] Bauer, JJ; Connelly, RR; Seterhenn, IA; Deausen, J; Srivastava, S; McLeod, DG; Moul, JW. Biostatistical modeling using traditional preoperative and pathological prognostic variables in the selection of men at high risk for disease recurrence after radical prostatectomy for prostate cancer. *J Urol,* 1998, 159, 929-933.
[251] D'Amico, AV; Whittington, R; Malkowicz, SB; Fondurulia, J; Chen, MH; Kaplan, I; Beard, CJ; Tomaszewski, JE; Renshaw, AA; Wein, A; Coleman, CN. Pretreatment nomogram for prostate-specific anti-genrecurrence after radical prostatectomy or external-beam radiation therapy for clinically localized prostate cancer. *J Clin Oncol.,* 1999, 17, 168-172.

[252] Moul, JW; Connelly, RR; Lubeck, DP; Bauer, JJ; Sun, L; Flanders, SC; Grossfeld, GD; Carroll, PR. Predicting risk of prostate specific antigen recurrence after radical prostatectomy with the Center for Prostate Disease Research and Cancer of the Prostate Strategic Urologic Research Endeavor databases. *J Urol.,* 2001, 166, 1322-1327.

[253] D'Amico, AV; Moul, JW; Carroll, PR; Sun, L; Lubeck, D; Chen, MH. Surrogate end point for prostate cancer-specific mortality after radical prostatectomy or radiation therapy. *J Natl Cancer Inst,* 2003, 95, 1376-1383.

[254] Patel, A; Dorey, F; Franklin, J; deKernion, JB. Recurrence patterns after radical retropubic prostatectomy: clinical usefulness of prostate specific antigen doubling times and log slope prostate specific antigen. *J Urol,* 1997, 158, 1441-1445.

[255] Soergel, TM; Koch, MO; Foster, RS; Bihrle, R; Wahle, G; Gardner, T; Jung, SH. Accuracy of predicting long-term prostate specific antigen outcome based on early prostate specific antigen recurrence results after radical prostatectomy. *J Urol* 2001, 166, 2198-2201.

[256] Terris, MK; Klonecke, AS; McDougall, IR; Stamey, TA. Utilization of bone scans in conjunction with prostate-specific antigen levels in the surveillance for recurrence of adenocarcinoma after radical prostatectomy. *J Nucl Med.,* 1991, 32, 1713-1717.

[257] Kahn, D; Williams, RD; Seldin, DW; Libertino, JA; Hirschhorn, M; Dreicer, R; Weiner, GJ; Bushnell, D; Gulfo, J. Radioimmunoscintigraphy with 111indium labeled CYT-356 for the detection of occult prostate cancer recurrence. *J Urol.,* 1994, 152, 1490-1495.

[258] http://www.ahrq.gov/clinic/uspstf08/prostate.

[259] http://www.aafp.org/online.

[260] 260.http://www.cancer.

[261] Lim, LS; Sherin, K. Screening for prostate cancer in U.S. men ACPM position statement on preventive practice. *Am J Prev Med,* 2008, 34, 164-170.

[262] Cooner, WH; Mosley, BR; Rutherford, CL; Jr., Beard, JH; Pond, HS; Bass, RB; Jr; Terry, WJ. Clinical application of transrectal ultrasonography and prostate specific antigen in the search for prostate cancer. *J Urol,* 1988, 139, 758-761.

[263] Brawer, MK. Prostate-specific antigen: current status. *CA Cancer J Clin,* 1999, 49, 264-281.

[264] Krumholtz, JS; Carvalhal, GF; Ramos, CG; Smith, DS; Thorson, P; Yan, Y; Humphrey, PA; Roehl, KA; Catalona WJ. Prostate-specific antigen cutoff of 2.6 ng/mL for prostate cancer screening is associated with favorable pathologic tumor features. *Urology,* 2002, 60, 469-473, discussion 473-464.

[265] Etzioni, R; Penson, DF; Legler, JM; di Tommaso, D; Boer, R; Gann, PH; Feuer, EJ. Overdiagnosis due to prostate-specific antigen screening: lessons from U.S. prostate cancer incidence trends. *J Natl Cancer Inst,* 2002, 94, 981-990.

[266] Punglia, RS; D'Amico, AV; Catalona, WJ; Roehl, KA; Kuntz, KM. Effect of verification bias on screening for prostate cancer by measurement of prostate-specific antigen. *N Engl J Med,* 2003, 349, 335-342.

[267] Stamey, TA; Caldwell, M; McNeal, JE; Nolley, R; Hemenez, M; Downs, J. The prostate specific antigen era in the United States is over for prostate cancer: what happened in the last 20 years? *J Urol,* 2004, 172, 1297-1301.

[268] Antenor, JA; Roehl, KA; Eggener, SE; Kundu, SD; Han, M; Catalona, WJ. Preoperative PSA and progression-free survival after radical prostatectomy for Stage T1c disease. *Urology,* 2005, 66, 156-160.

[269] Freedland, SJ; Mangold, LA; Walsh, PC; Partin, AW. The prostatic specific antigen era is alive and well: prostatic specific antigen and biochemical progression following radical prostatectomy. *J Urol,* 2005, 174, 1276-1281, discussion 1281, author reply 1281.

[270] Essink-Bot, ML; de Koning, HJ; Nijs, HG; Kirkels, WJ; van der Maas, PJ; Schroder, FH. Short-term effects of population-based screening for prostate cancer on health-related quality of life. *J Natl Cancer Inst.,* 1998, 90, 925-931.

[271] Labrie, F; Candas, B; Cusan, L; Gomez, JL; Belanger, A; Brousseau, G; Chevrette, E; Levesque, J. Screening decreases prostate cancer mortality: 11-year follow-up of the 1988 Quebec prospective randomized controlled trial. *Prostate,* 2004, 59, 311-318.

[272] Schroder, FH; Hugosson, J; Roobol, MJ; Tammela, TL; Ciatto, S; Nelen, V; Kwiatkowski, M; Lujan, M; Lilja, H; Zappa, M; Denis, LJ; Recker, F; Berenguer, A; Maattanen, L; Bangma, CH; Aus, G; Villers, A; Rebillard, X; van der Kwast, T; Blijenberg, BG; Moss, SM; de Koning, HJ; Auvinen, A. Screening and prostate-cancer mortality in a randomized European study. *N Engl J Med.,* 2009, 360, 1320-1328.

[273] Walsh, PC. Mortality results form a randomized prostate-cancer screening trial. *The Journal of Urology.,* 2009, 182, 146-147.
[274] Walsh, PC. Screening and prostate cancer mortality in a randomized european study. *The Journal of Urology.,* 2009, 145-146.
[275] Wilt, TJ; Brawer, MK; Barry, MJ; Jones, KM; Kwon, Y; Gingrich, JR; Aronson, WJ; Nsouli, I; Iyer, P; Cartagena, R; Snider, G; Roehrborn, C; Fox, S. The Prostate cancer Intervention Versus Observation Trial:VA/NCI/AHRQ Cooperative Studies Program #407 (PIVOT): design and baseline results of a randomized controlled trial comparing radical prostatectomy to watchful waiting for men with clinically localized prostate cancer. *Contemp Clin Trials.,* 2009, 30, 81-87.
[276] Donovan, J; Hamdy, F; Neal, D; Peters, T; Oliver, S; Brindle, L; Jewell, D; Powell, P; Gillatt, D; Dedman, D; Mills, N; Smith, M; Noble, S; Lane, A. Prostate Testing for Cancer and Treatment (ProtecT) feasibility study. *Health Technol Assess.,* 2003, 7, 1-88.

Index

A

absorption, 9
absorption coefficient, 9
access, 7
accuracy, 2, 17
acid, vii, 1, 3, 4, 6, 7, 18, 30, 34, 36, 52
activation, 6, 8, 9, 13, 35, 40, 41
active site, 7
adenocarcinoma, 32, 45, 48, 49, 53
adhesion, 40
administration, 1
advancement, 16, 18
AF, 39, 45
African American, 20
age, vii, 1, 10, 11, 12, 13, 15, 20, 21, 23, 29, 42, 43, 44, 45, 47
agent, 37
aggressiveness, 52
aid, 50
AJ, 43, 46
AL, 49, 51
alpha, 30, 36, 37, 42, 43, 44
alternative, 17, 25, 34
alternatives, 21
alters, 10
American Cancer Society, 20, 42, 45
amino, vii, 6, 7, 8, 13, 34
amino acid, vii, 6, 7, 8, 13
amino acids, vii, 6, 7, 8, 13
androgen, 5, 9, 33, 34, 40
androgens, 1, 5
angiogenesis, 18
angiogenic, 9
Antibodies, 8
antibody, 4, 7, 17, 36, 47
antigen, vii, 1, 2, 3, 4, 17, 18, 30, 31, 32, 33, 34, 35, 36, 37, 38, 39, 40, 41, 42, 43, 44, 45, 46, 47, 48, 49, 50, 51, 52, 53, 54
antitumor, 9
AP, 32, 46
apoptosis, 51
apoptotic, 41
arginine, 6
argument, 22
assessment, 20, 31

B

back, 18
base, 43, 47, 48, 50, 54
bcl-2, 51
beam radiation, 31, 51, 52
behavior, 6
benefits, vii, 2, 20, 21, 22, 49
benign, vii, 2, 3, 4, 8, 14, 17, 30, 31, 32, 33, 37, 38, 40, 41, 42, 43, 45, 49, 52
benign prostatic hyperplasia, 8, 37, 38, 40, 41, 42, 52
benign prostatic hypertrophy, 31
bias, 22, 54
binding, 6, 7, 9, 18, 36, 39, 40

biochemistry, 37
biomarker, 5, 10, 17
biomarkers, 2, 5, 16, 18, 43, 50, 51, 52
biopsies, 12, 15, 39, 42, 45, 46, 47
biopsy, vii, 9, 10, 11, 12, 13, 15, 16, 17, 20, 21, 22, 23, 24, 45
blood, 5, 7, 10, 12, 39, 41
blot, 37, 49
body fluid, 3, 4, 16, 33
bonds, 6, 7, 8
bone, 1, 9, 19, 53
bone scan, 19, 53
boys, 42
brachytherapy, 18
bradykinin, 5
breast cancer, 10, 40, 41

C

calibration, 39
calmodulin, 41
cAMP, 40
cancer, vii, 1, 2, 4, 9, 10, 11, 12, 14, 16, 20, 22, 23, 24, 29, 30, 31, 32, 33, 34, 35, 36, 38, 40, 41, 42, 43, 44, 45, 46, 47, 48, 49, 50, 51, 52, 53, 54, 55
cancer cells, 41
cancer screening, 23, 24, 30, 44, 54
candidates, 19
carbohydrate, 35
carcinoma, 13, 14, 37, 43, 46, 52
castration, 1, 9
cDNA, 6, 34
CE, 46
cell, 9, 40
cell adhesion, 40
cell line, 40
cell lines, 40
cell surface, 9
chromosome, vii, 5, 32, 48
chymotrypsin, 7, 36
CL, 34, 35, 38, 47, 50, 53
cleavage, 6, 8, 9, 38
clinical application, 25, 52
clinical trial, 23, 30, 43, 44

clinically significant, 22
clinics, 14, 19
cloning, 34
coagulation, 32
coagulum, vii, 9
coding, 32, 34
community, vii, 43, 46, 47
compliance, 23
complications, 1
composition, 7
concentration, 5, 41, 42
Congress, iv
consensus, vii, 9, 13, 25
control, 11, 23, 24, 43, 50
control group, 23, 24
controversial, 25
controversies, 15, 21
conversion, 35
correlation, 9, 22, 40
cost, 13, 15, 24
cost effectiveness, 24
counsel, 21
covalent, 7
CPT, 16
CR, 50, 51
cryotherapy, 19
crystal structure, 7
CT, 19
CT scan, 19

D

death, 19, 23, 24, 31, 41
deaths, 1, 19
degradation, 36
density, vii, 2, 12, 14, 30, 44, 45, 46, 47
derivatives, 16
detectable, 10, 13
detection, vii, 1, 2, 3, 4, 11, 15, 16, 17, 19, 20, 21, 22, 23, 24, 25, 30, 38, 42, 43, 44, 45, 46, 47, 48, 53
dietary, 1
differentiation, 35, 43, 45
digestion, 6
Discovery, vii

Index

discriminatory, 22
diseases, 2, 8, 10
disulfide, 8
disulfide bonds, 8
DNA, 18
DNA ploidy, 18
drug treatment, 10
drugs, 10

E

EB, 50, 51
Education, 43
ejaculation, 9, 10, 41
elderly, 1
electrophoresis, 4, 6
EM, 51
encoding, 34
endometrium, 5, 33
endoplasmic reticulum, 6
enlargement, 11, 49
environment, 5
environmental factors, 1, 29
enzymatic, 5, 7, 9, 16
enzymatic activity, 5, 7, 9, 16
enzyme, 7, 32, 49
enzyme immunoassay, 32
enzyme-linked immunosorbent assay, 49
enzymes, 35, 37
epithelial cell, 5, 17
epithelial cells, 5, 17
epithelium, 5, 15, 37
epitope, 8
epitopes, 8
ER, 6
ET, 31
ethnicity, 29
evidence, vii, 3, 4, 8, 10, 14, 16, 17, 19, 20, 21, 31, 33

F

failure, 18, 19, 23, 51
false negative, 21

false positive, 2, 11, 16, 20, 21
family, vii, 1, 5, 7, 20, 21, 29, 32, 37
family history, 1, 20, 21, 29
family physician, 20
FD, 29
FDA, 1, 4, 8, 10, 12
fibroblast, 9
fibroblast growth factor, 9
fibronectin, 9
financial, 12
first degree relative, 20
fluid, 5, 10, 17, 35, 50
fluorescence, 50
Ford, 47
formation, 6, 37, 38
Fox, 55
FP, 31
fragments, 8, 9
FS, 32
functional analysis, 48

G

GE, 51
gel, 4, 6
gelation, 39
gene, 5, 17, 31, 32, 34, 48, 49, 52
gene expression, 17, 49, 52
generation, 9
genes, 5, 32, 34
genome, 5, 16
GH, 42, 47
GL, 30, 32, 42, 46
gland, 5, 7, 41
glycoprotein, 17, 35
glycoproteins, 6
glycosylation, 35
gold, 33
groups, 1, 3, 6, 8, 15, 23
growth, 9, 14, 18, 19, 39, 40, 48
growth factor, 9, 18, 39, 40
growth rate, 14
guidelines, 19, 20, 24

H

HA, 33, 34, 39, 41, 42, 44, 46, 47, 48
harm, 20
health, vii, 20, 21, 23, 54
health care, 20, 21
health care professionals, 20
hemostasis, 5
high risk, 20, 21, 51, 52
histological, 1
histological examination, 1
history, 1, 20, 21, 29, 51
homology, 5, 7, 16, 36
horizon, 49
hormonal therapy, 1, 19
hormone, 9, 40
hormones, 29
human, 3, 4, 5, 7, 9, 16, 18, 29, 31, 32, 33, 34, 35, 36, 37, 39, 41, 45, 47, 48
human body, 7, 9, 18
human genome, 5, 16
humans, vii, 3
hydrogen, 7
hydrogen bonds, 7
hyperplasia, 8, 37, 38, 40, 41, 42, 45, 52
hypertrophy, 31

I

IB, 33
ideal, 21, 50
identification, 31, 39
identity, 31
IGF, 9
IGF-1, 9
imaging, 17, 19
immunoassays, 38, 39
immunohistochemical, 37
immunological, 3
implementation, 19
in vitro, 37
in vivo, 9
inactivation, 9, 40
inactive, 6, 7, 8, 9, 12, 37
incidence, vii, 11, 42, 54
inclusion, 14
indication, 15
indium, 19
induction, 33
infertility, 3
inflammation, 10, 34
inhibitor, 7, 9, 36, 37, 42
inhibitors, 7, 10, 12, 13, 36, 37
injury, iv, 10
insulin, 9, 39, 40
Insulin like growth factor, 18
insulin-like growth factor, 39, 40
international standards, 39
interval, 19, 20, 23, 46
investigative, 44
IR, 53
IRP, 9
IS, 30, 46
isoleucine, 6
issues, 13, 20

J

JAMA, 30, 31, 43, 44, 45, 47, 51
Japanese, 3
JI, 45, 50, 51
JT, 29, 38, 41, 46, 51, 52
Jung, 39, 48, 49, 53

K

Ki-67, 52
kinetics, 19
kinins, 32

L

LA, 29, 30, 31, 32, 33, 41, 42, 47, 49, 51, 54
labeling, 45
LC, 29, 39
lead, 11, 22
leakage, 10
leucine, 6

life expectancy, 19, 20
limitation, 21, 24
limitations, 20, 21, 24, 38
linear, 19
liquefaction, 9, 39
liver, 5
LM, 47
localization, 33
long period, 14
Luo, 32
lymph, 17, 48, 49
lymph node, 17, 48, 49

M

majority, 13, 23
males, 4, 5, 11, 15
malignancy, 1
malignant, 3, 4, 5, 8, 31, 33, 38
malignant tumors, 33
mammalian cell, 35
mammalian cells, 35
man, 23
management, 46
manipulation, 10, 41
mask, 8
mass, 6, 9, 13, 35, 44
mass spectrometry, 6, 9, 13, 44
matter, 3
MB, 41
measurement, 9, 14, 15, 38, 43, 47, 54
measurements, vii, 2, 5, 12, 14, 30, 38
measures, 19, 45
median, 23
medical, 1, 2, 21
men, 1, 2, 4, 5, 12, 14, 15, 19, 20, 23, 24, 30, 37, 41, 42, 44, 45, 46, 47, 48, 51, 52, 53, 55
messenger RNA, 41
metastases, 48, 49, 51
metastasis, 4, 9, 17, 52
metastatic, 18
metastatic disease, 18
migration, 2, 11, 19, 25
MIT, 31

mitogen, 9
ML, 50, 51, 54
modalities, 1
modality, 19
modeling, 52
models, 7
modulation, 9, 40
molecular biology, 34
molecular mass, 6, 9
molecular weight, vii, 4, 5, 17
monoclonal, 7, 8, 16, 17, 37, 47
monoclonal antibodies, 8, 16, 37, 47
Monoclonal antibodies, 31
monoclonal antibody, 7, 17
morbidity, vii, 21
mortality, vii, 1, 2, 19, 20, 21, 23, 24, 25, 42, 51, 53, 54, 55
mouse, 40
mRNA, 6, 32, 33

N

national community, 43
neoplasia, 47, 49
network, 48
neural network, 48
normal, 3, 5, 9, 10, 17, 31, 37, 42
nuclear, 48

O

observations, 39
old age, 15
oligosaccharide, 6
Oncology, 18
online, 53
operator, 17
organ, 18, 48
osteoblasts, 40

P

p53, 18, 51
PA, 8, 30, 33, 36, 37, 39, 43, 48, 51, 54

parameter, 46
parathyroid, 9, 40
parathyroid hormone, 9, 40
Parnes, 47
participants, 23
patients, 1, 4, 8, 9, 10, 11, 12, 13, 14, 15, 17, 18, 19, 20, 21, 22, 23, 25, 30, 31, 37, 40, 41, 44, 49, 51
PCA, 17
PE, 32, 34, 39
peptide, 6, 9, 41
PF, 30, 42, 50
physical activity, 10
physiological, 14
Physiological, 45
placenta, 5
plasma, vii, 3, 4, 5, 6, 7, 31, 32, 35, 37, 38, 39, 41, 43
plasma membrane, 6
plasminogen, 9, 35, 37
play, 9, 13
population, 11, 14, 15, 21, 23, 24, 43, 45, 47, 54
potential benefits, 20
power, 22
prediction, 2, 14, 22, 25, 43
predictors, 46, 47
preparation, iv
prevention, 16
preventive, 53
prodrugs, 10
production, 40
professionals, 2, 20, 21
prognosis, 4, 16, 17, 25, 50
prognostic marker, 52
program, 43
proliferation, 9
promoter, 6, 34
promoter region, 6, 34
prostate cancer, 2, 9, 20, 23, 24, 29, 30, 31, 32, 33, 34, 35, 36, 38, 40, 41, 42, 43, 44, 45, 46, 47, 48, 49, 50, 51, 52, 53, 54, 55
Prostate cancer, vii, 1, 29, 30, 46, 55
prostate carcinoma, 13, 14, 37, 43, 52
prostate gland, 5, 7, 41
prostate specific antigen, vii, 1, 3, 4, 30, 31, 33, 34, 35, 36, 38, 39, 40, 41, 43, 44, 45, 46, 49, 50, 53, 54
prostatectomy, 4, 5, 18, 19, 22, 33, 50, 51, 52, 53, 54, 55
prostatitis, 10, 20
protease inhibitors, 7, 12, 13, 37
proteases, 5, 7, 34
protein, 3, 4, 5, 6, 7, 9, 17, 31, 33, 35, 37, 39, 40, 48
proteinase, 36, 38
proteins, 3, 4, 5, 6, 17, 18, 39, 51
proteolysis, 40
proteolytic enzyme, 35
proteomics, 16
protocol, 17
protocols, 9
PSA, vii, 1, 2, 3, 4, 5, 6, 7, 8, 9, 10, 11, 12, 13, 14, 15, 16, 17, 18, 19, 20, 21, 22, 23, 25, 30, 31, 34, 35, 36, 37, 38, 39, 40, 41, 42, 44, 45, 46, 47, 48, 50, 51, 54
PT, 30, 38, 42, 43, 47, 52
puberty, 10, 42
purification, 16, 31

Q

quality assurance, 38
quality of life, 54
Quebec, 54

R

RA, 29, 42, 45, 50
race, 1, 18, 20, 21
radiation, 1, 31, 51, 52, 53
radiation therapy, 31, 52, 53
radiotherapy, 18, 19
ramp, 44
range, 2, 5, 12, 13, 14, 16, 45, 47
rape, 3
RB, 30, 42, 43, 44, 53
RC, 30, 38, 42, 45, 47, 49
reactions, 36, 39

Index

reactivity, 8, 47
reading, 27
reagents, 39
receptors, 9, 40
recognition, 8
recommendations, vii, 8, 15, 19, 20, 21
rectal examination, vii, 1, 10, 30, 42, 43, 45, 47, 50
recurrence, vii, 5, 18, 22, 25, 50, 51, 52, 53
refractory, 40
regulation, 32, 34, 36, 37
relationship, 14
relatives, 20
resistance, 13
response, 34, 40
reticulum, 6
risk, 1, 11, 12, 16, 18, 20, 21, 22, 29, 31, 40, 46, 51, 52, 53
risk assessment, 20
risk factors, 1, 51
RNA, 17, 41, 50
Rutherford, 53

S

safety, 42
sample, 39
sampling, 46
scientific community, vii
scope, 18
SD, 35, 37, 38, 40, 47, 49, 54
SDS, 8
SE, 51, 54
search, 53
secrete, 39
secretion, 6, 33
sediments, 50
semen, 3, 4, 9, 31, 37, 39
seminal vesicle, 35, 37, 45
sensitivity, vii, 2, 15, 16, 21, 22, 30, 45
series, 42
serine, 5, 6, 7, 34, 35, 36, 48
serum, vii, 1, 2, 4, 5, 6, 7, 8, 10, 11, 12, 13, 14, 15, 16, 17, 18, 22, 25, 30, 31, 32, 35, 36, 37, 38, 39, 40, 41, 42, 43, 44, 45, 46, 47, 48, 49, 50
sex, 39
shape, 15, 38
shares, 7, 16
short period, 14
Short-term, 54
signal peptide, 6
similarity, 34
single chain, 38
sites, 7
skeletal muscle, 48
society, 10
species, 33
specificity, vii, 2, 7, 12, 13, 14, 15, 16, 21, 22, 30, 36, 44, 45
sperm, 3, 9
spermatozoa, 39
SR, 41
stability, 7
stages, 11
standardization, 8, 38, 39
standards, 39
Standards, 8, 39
states, 20
statistics, 29
Steroid, 34
steroids, 6, 40
structure, vii, 7, 8, 32, 35, 36, 38, 39
substrate, 7, 36
suffering, 16, 17, 20
Sun, 53
surgery, 1
surveillance, 42, 53
survival, 2, 24, 25, 42, 54
survival rate, 42
sweat, 5
symptoms, 1

T

tamoxifen, 40
target, 36
targets, 49
techniques, 3, 4, 16

technologies, 18
ternary complex, 36
testing, 5, 17, 19, 21, 23, 30
testosterone, 11
TGF, 40
therapeutic use, 10
therapy, 1, 18, 23, 29, 31, 36, 49, 51, 52, 53
threshold, vii, 1, 2, 10, 11, 13, 14, 15, 16, 21, 22, 23
thymidine, 45
thyroid, 5
tissue, 1, 3, 4, 5, 6, 10, 16, 17, 31, 32, 34, 37, 38, 49, 52
trans, 6
transcript, 34
transcriptional, 34
transforming growth factor, 9
transition, 37, 38, 46
trauma, 12, 20
treatment, 1, 2, 3, 10, 11, 18, 19, 20
trial, 11, 16, 23, 24, 30, 42, 43, 44, 54, 55
trust, 19
trypsin, 7, 8, 16, 35
tumor, 1, 4, 10, 11, 15, 16, 18, 21, 22, 24, 34, 40, 45, 49, 51, 54
tumor progression, 40
tumors, 2, 5, 8, 16, 18, 22, 30, 33, 41, 48, 49

U

ultrasonography, 14, 19, 45, 53
ultrasound, 15
uniform, 24, 39
United, 1, 20, 22, 23, 24, 42, 54
United Kingdom, 24
United States, 1, 20, 22, 23, 42, 54
urethra, 5
urinary, 5, 33, 50
urine, 17, 50
urokinase, 35
urology, 19, 46

V

validation, 50
valuation, 44
values, vii, 2, 5, 8, 12, 13, 15, 16, 20, 21, 22, 47
variability, 8, 14, 15, 46
variables, 18, 51, 52
variation, 45
vascular endothelial growth factor, 9
VC, 31, 43
velocity, vii, 2, 13, 31, 45, 46, 51
vesicle, 35, 39, 45
vesicles, 6, 37
viscosity, 9

W

Weinberg, 45
Western blot, 37, 49
women, 41
World Health Organization (WHO), 9, 39
WP, 34, 50

X

xenografts, 41

Y

yield, 42

Z

zinc, 7
Zn, 36